Praise for *Critical Conversations in Healthcare,* 3rd Edition

"*Critical Conversations in Healthcare, 3rd Edition,* imparts useful tools and resources to enhance effective communication using not only verbal means but also other influences including body language, tone, and mindfulness. Cheri's approach enables the reader to pause, take a breath, lean in, and listen with clarity and confidence. Regardless of position or title, healthcare professionals from the bedside to the boardroom will discover* Critical Conversations in Healthcare *as a complement to enhance competency and purpose in managing communication to promote 'win-win' results."*

–Martin S. Manno, PhD, RN, NEA-BC, CEN
Associate Chief Nurse, Medical Center Education and Library Services
Corporal Michael J. Crescenz VA Medical Center
Philadelphia, PA

"*Cheri Clancy's* Critical Conversations in Healthcare *is a superb and inclusive primer on the importance of communication skills for practicing nurses. It covers multiple frameworks including emotional intelligence and competence as they inform interpersonal skills development and execution, often in difficult circumstances. This well-crafted translational work is organized around practical guidelines and application of effective, actionable techniques across contexts, including organizational culture and behavior. It is a wonderful resource on conversational know-how in healthcare."*

–Joan Kearney, PhD, APRN, FAAN
Professor and Chair, Yale University School of Nursing

"*Cheri Clancy delivers once more with this essential guide for healthcare professionals navigating intricate conversations. Packed with practical insights and strategies, this book empowers readers to communicate effectively and compassionately in difficult scenarios, ultimately enhancing patient outcomes and interprofessional relationships."*

–Bob Dent, DNP, RN, FACHE, FAAN, FAONL
Chief Nursing Officer, Emory Healthcare
President, Dr. Bob Dent, LLC

"The third edition of Critical Conversations in Healthcare could not have been more timely. The pandemic and its aftermath, compounded by the social and political polarization of recent years, have made meaningful conversations both more important and more challenging than ever before. This book offers a complete and easy-to-follow formula for choosing the right words, right tone, and right body language for every situation. Thoroughly researched and documented yet easy to use, this is a must-read for everyone in a healthcare leadership role."

–Joe Tye, MHA, MBA
Consultant, speaker, and author
Adjunct Assistant Professor, University of Iowa College of
Public Health's Department of Health Management and Policy

"Cheri Clancy has done it again. In her third edition of Critical Conversations in Healthcare, Clancy offers great insights and practical tools for elevating communications at all levels. Whether managing conflict, doing service recovery, or leading change, Clancy presents excellent, easy-to-implement tools for effective and empathetic communication. She clearly understands the nuances of healthcare communication and what it takes to build a culture that fosters open, respectful, and clear communication. This book is applicable to a broad range of readers, from early-career professionals wanting to develop new skills to senior executives who want to elevate relationships."

–Kristin Baird, MHA, BSN
President/CEO, Baird Group

"Cheri Clancy has written a book with invaluable advice to guide readers in communicating with colleagues and patients professionally, thoughtfully, and empathetically. She carefully provides a road map to guide good communication in conversations and situations frequently encountered in practice. Critical Conversations in Healthcare is a book that will facilitate meaningful discourse leading to better patient care and careers characterized by impactful and meaningful conversations."

–Marie O'Toole, EdD, RN, FAAN, ANEF
Professor & Senior Associate Dean for Academic and Faculty Affairs
Camden School of Nursing, Rutgers University

"A must-read for any healthcare professional. This is a fantastic depiction of how positive communication is multifaceted. It plays an integral part in our personal, professional, and patient relationships."

–Stephanie Ferroni, PMHNP
Cooper Care Alliance Department of Psychiatry
Cooper Health

THIRD EDITION

CRITICAL CONVERSATIONS IN HEALTHCARE

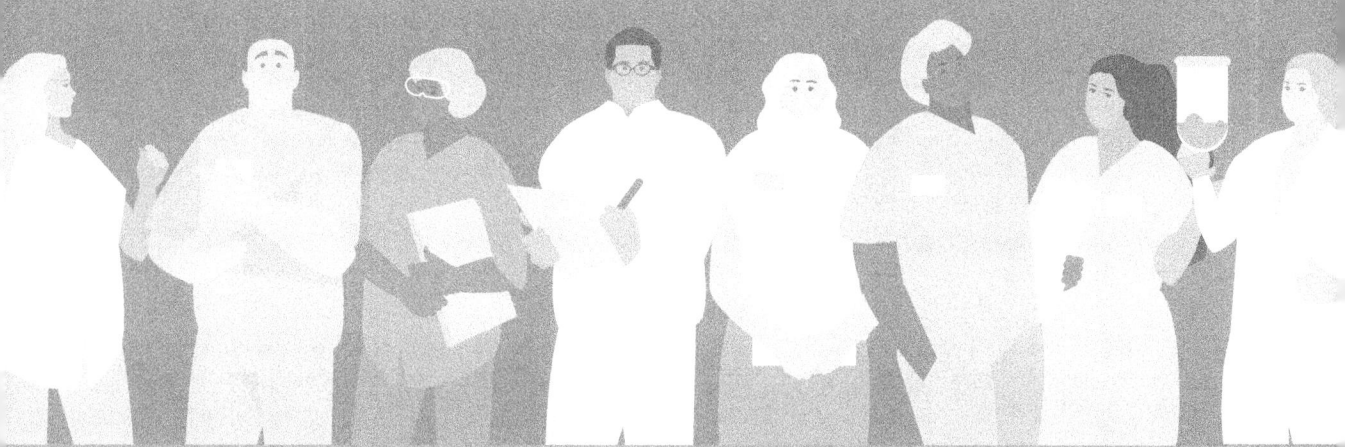

Scripts & Techniques for Effective Interprofessional & Patient Communication

Cheri Clancy, MSN, MS, RN, NEA-BC, CPXP

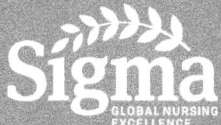

Copyright © 2024 by Sigma Theta Tau International Honor Society of Nursing

All rights reserved. This book is protected by copyright. No part of it may be reproduced, stored in a retrieval system, or transmitted in any form or by any means, electronic, mechanical, photocopying, recording, or otherwise, without written permission from the publisher. Any trademarks, service marks, design rights, or similar rights that are mentioned, used, or cited in this book are the property of their respective owners. Their use here does not imply that you may use them for a similar or any other purpose.

This book is not intended to be a substitute for the medical advice of a licensed medical professional. The author and publisher have made every effort to ensure the accuracy of the information contained within at the time of its publication and shall have no liability or responsibility to any person or entity regarding any loss or damage incurred, or alleged to have incurred, directly or indirectly, by the information contained in this book. The author and publisher make no warranties, express or implied, with respect to its content, and no warranties may be created or extended by sales representatives or written sales materials. The author and publisher have no responsibility for the consistency or accuracy of URLs and content of third-party websites referenced in this book.

Sigma Theta Tau International Honor Society of Nursing (Sigma) is a nonprofit organization whose mission is developing nurse leaders anywhere to improve healthcare everywhere. Founded in 1922, Sigma has more than 135,000 active members in over 100 countries and territories. Members include practicing nurses, instructors, researchers, policymakers, entrepreneurs, and others. Sigma's more than 540 chapters are located at more than 700 institutions of higher education throughout Armenia, Australia, Botswana, Brazil, Canada, Chile, Colombia, Croatia, England, Eswatini, Finland, Ghana, Hong Kong, Ireland, Israel, Italy, Jamaica, Japan, Jordan, Kenya, Lebanon, Malawi, Mexico, the Netherlands, Nigeria, Pakistan, Philippines, Portugal, Puerto Rico, Scotland, Singapore, South Africa, South Korea, Sweden, Taiwan, Tanzania, Thailand, the United States, and Wales. Learn more at www.sigmanursing.org.

Sigma Theta Tau International
550 West North Street
Indianapolis, IN, USA 46202

To request a review copy for course adoption, order additional books, buy in bulk, or purchase for corporate use, contact Sigma Marketplace at 888.654.4968 (US/Canada toll-free), +1.317.687.2256 (International), or solutions@sigmamarketplace.org.

To request author information, or for speaker or other media requests, contact Sigma Marketing at 888.634.7575 (US/Canada toll-free) or +1.317.634.8171 (International).

ISBN: 9781646481934
EPUB ISBN: 9781646481941
PDF ISBN: 9781646481958

Library of Congress Cataloging-in-Publication Data

Names: Clancy, Cheri, 1972- author. | Sigma Theta Tau International, issuing body.

Title: Critical conversations in healthcare : scripts & techniques for effective interprofessional & patient communication / Cheri Clancy.

Description: Third edition. | Indianapolis, IN : Sigma Theta Tau International Honor Society of Nursing, [2024] | Includes bibliographical references and index. | Summary: "This book reveals the key factors behind how others perceive us when we communicate with them-things like attitude, body language, and word choice. But it goes even further to discuss the neurochemicals that drive these perceptions.

Understanding all these different factors can help us approach conversations and communications with openness to promote superior outcomes. Armed with the knowledge and skills you'll gain from reading this book, you'll be able to quickly identify when a conversation isn't going the way you intended and get things back on track"-- Provided by publisher.

Identifiers: LCCN 2024013934 (print) | LCCN 2024013935 (ebook) | ISBN 9781646481934 (paperback) | ISBN 9781646481941 (epub) | ISBN 9781646481958 (PDF)

Subjects: MESH: Nurse-Patient Relations | Health Communication | Interprofessional Relations

Classification: LCC RA423.2 (print) | LCC RA423.2 (ebook) | NLM WY 88 | DDC 362.101/4--dc23/eng/20240408

LC record available at https://lccn.loc.gov/2024013934

LC ebook record available at https://lccn.loc.gov/2024013935

Publisher: Dustin Sullivan
Acquisitions Editor: Emily Hatch
Project Editor: Todd Lothery
Cover Designer: Rebecca Batchelor
Interior Design/Page Layout: Rebecca Batchelor
Indexer: Larry Sweazy

Managing Editor: Carla Hall
Publications Specialist: Todd Lothery
Development Editor: Jillmarie Leeper Sycamore
Copy Editor: Todd Lothery
Proofreader: Erin Geile
Illustrator: Malcolm Ribot

Dedication

This book is dedicated to:

My three beautiful children: Paige, Shane, and Colin. "I love you more…."

My husband, family, and friends, for your unconditional love, support, and laughter.

Everyone working in the healthcare field, for committing your life to caring for others.

–Cheri Clancy

Acknowledgments

A special thank you to Carla Hall, Emily Hatch, Todd Lothery, and Jillmarie Leeper Sycamore of Sigma Theta Tau International for helping me to bring education, insight, and excellence to this book. I am so appreciative for all of your support and guidance.

Thank you to Dr. Shelley Johnson for your contributions to Chapter 10 and your genuine friendship and mentorship over the years.

About the Author

Cheri Clancy, MSN, MS, RN, NEA-BC, CPXP, is a board-certified ANCC nurse executive with more than 20 years of leadership experience. She earned a bachelor of science in nursing from Thomas Jefferson University and a master of science in health administration and wellness promotion from California College for Health Sciences as well as a master of science in nursing in organizational leadership from Independence University. Clancy also completed the Wharton Executive Leadership Program at the University of Pennsylvania in 2014.

Clancy is the founder of Cheri Clancy & Associates, LLC, a coaching and training firm that uses hard science as a catalyst for soft-skill leadership development. Areas of specialty include patient-experience strategy, empathy training, critical conversations, and building workplace resiliency. She is committed to helping organizations build healthy and productive workplace environments. In addition to presenting, coaching, and consulting, Clancy also leads the client experience department at Bayada Home Health Agency.

Clancy is a member of many professional organizations, including the New Jersey State Nurses Association (NJSNA), the American Nurses Association (ANA), the Beryl Institute, the American Organization of Nurse Leaders (AONL), Sigma Theta Tau International Honor Society of Nursing (Sigma), and the Organization of Nurse Leaders, New Jersey (ONL NJ).

Clancy has received various honors and awards. In 2015 she was featured as the "Leader to Watch" in the AONL *Voice of Nursing Leadership* journal. In 2016 she received the Professional Nurse Recognition Award from ONL NJ, and in 2018 she received the Nursing Beacon of Light Award from the NJSNA.

About the Contributing Author (Chapter 10)

Shelley A. Johnson, EdD, RN, received her baccalaureate degree from the University of Pennsylvania School of Nursing, a master of science from Pennsylvania State University, and a doctorate in educational leadership from the University of Phoenix. She also holds certificates from Harvard University in educational leadership, the University of Pennsylvania in community participatory research, and in diversity, equity, and inclusion.

Johnson has taught and led undergraduate and graduate programs for more than 20 years. She has worked in higher education leadership for Chamberlain University, University of Phoenix, Rutgers University, LaSalle University, and University of Medicine and Dentistry of New Jersey.

She was the founding Director and Chair of Nursing and Health Science at Lincoln University in Pennsylvania. She has served as a Dean at Chamberlain University and as an independent consultant via Kairos Solutions, LLC. Her specialties include higher education, leadership, curriculum and instruction, assessment, and community health. She is certified as a nurse executive, nurse educator, and comprehensive systematic reviewer. Currently, Johnson serves as University Provost for Salem University.

Johnson practices servant leadership. She is president of Sigma Theta Tau, Xi Chapter, at the University of Pennsylvania, and serves on other community organization boards. She has published articles and contributed chapters to various books, served as a subject matter expert, and participated in research related to a variety of topics, including perceptions of student bullying, health disparities, cultural diversity, advocacy, leadership, and nursing education. Research interests include nursing and general educational practices, healthy work environments, and leadership development. Johnson conducts presentations and workshops on these topics for educational and business groups.

Additional Book Resources

For additional resources for this book, including a sample chapter, visit this book's Sigma Repository page by using the link or QR code below.

https://sigma.nursingrepository.org/handle/10755/23599

Special Note to Readers

Here at Sigma, we realize that language is constantly evolving. The meaning of a word often changes over time, some words become obsolete, and some terms that were once acceptable may become controversial or even offensive, depending on the context or circumstances. We have made every effort to make language choices that are inclusive and not offensive. Should you identify words in this book that you believe negatively impact a group or groups of people, please reach out to us at Publications@SigmaNursing.org.

Table of Contents

About the Author...ix
Introduction..xvii

1 The Importance of Effective Communication in Healthcare .. 1
Hierarchy of Needs 3
In the Driver's Seat: Finding Common Sense in Not-So-Common Conversations 5
Understanding Your Own Social Style and Others'..8
The Benefits of Understanding the Social Styles in Healthcare 11
Taking the BEST Approach to Effective Conversations...16
Integrating Teach-Back Into Your Conversations..25
Your Road Map: Guiding Principles for Effective Communication.................................29
The Drive Home...31
References 32

2 Body Language Exposed 33
In the Driver's Seat: Understanding and Interpreting Body Language...........................35
How to Tell if Someone Isn't Being Honest With You 39
Your Road Map: Improving Body Language Messaging and Interpretation....................55
The Drive Home...61
References 62

3 The Emotionally Intelligent and Emotionally Competent Nurse 63
In the Driver's Seat: Understanding Your Emotions and Your Intelligence 66
Your Road Map: Improving Your EI and EC 73
The Drive Home...91
References 94

4 Mindful Conversations.. 97
In the Driver's Seat: Be Mindful, Not Mind Full 100
Your Road Map: Communicating Mindfully 105
The Drive Home...107
References 108

5	**Mind Over Matter** **109**
	In the Driver's Seat: The Science Behind Communication 111
	Your Road Map: Improving Your Mind to Improve Your Outcomes 116
	The Drive Home 120
	References 121

6	**Impromptu Scripting, Phrasing, and Acronyms** **123**
	In the Driver's Seat: Using Impromptu Scripts 125
	Your Road Map: Acronyms and Emotional Intelligence....................................... 126
	The Drive Home 140
	References 140

7	**Interprofessional Coaching Conversations** **141**
	In the Driver's Seat: How to Discuss What Matters Most 142
	Your Road Map: Applying the BEST Approach in Coaching Conversations 156
	The Drive Home 163
	References 163

8	**Improving Patient Experience** **165**
	In the Driver's Seat: Perception Is Reality 167
	Developing an Effective Patient Experience Strategy 167
	Your Road Map: Communicate, Communicate, Communicate........................... 176
	The Drive Home 188
	References 189

9	**Fostering a Healthy Workplace Environment** **191**
	In the Driver's Seat: Embracing Change 193
	Your Road Map: Building an HWE Starts With You 195
	The Drive Home 207
	References 208

10	**Organizational Culture and Behavior** **211**
	In the Driver's Seat: Defining Organizational Culture and Behavior.................. 212
	Your Road Map: Understanding Organizational Cultural and Behaviors 215
	Assessing and Improving Organizational Culture and Behavior 224
	The Drive Home 227
	References 227

11 On Social Media 229

The Pros of Social Media 230
Social Media for Healthcare Professionals: Networking and Staying Informed 230
Information Resources on the Web for Healthcare Professionals 233
Social Media as a Powerful Tool for Health Education and Promotion 235
The Cons of Social Media 238
Social Media for Healthcare Professionals: Navigating Ethical and Legal Issues 239
Doing Your Due Diligence 240
References 245

12 Conclusion 247

References 252

A Sample Rounding Template 253

Sample Transformational Rounding Template 254
Sample Rounding on Internal Departments 262
Reference 269

B Develop Your Own AIDET Worksheet 271

Index 275

Introduction

"I've learned that people will forget what you said, people will forget what you did, but people will never forget how you made them feel."
–Maya Angelou

When we experience flow in a conversation—when the conversation feels effortless and enjoyable—we leave feeling valued and respected. In these types of conversations, there's no sense of anxiety or awkwardness. Neither person feels stuck nor trapped. We are respectfully listening and responding to each other.

All too often, however, our conversations have a less positive outcome. For example, maybe you sense the other person has no idea or no interest in what you're talking about. Or maybe they become visibly upset or angry.

What causes these types of negative outcomes? Why is it—even when you have the best intentions—your conversations take a turn for the worse? And how can you prevent this from happening? That's what this book is about.

This book reveals the key factors behind how others perceive us when we communicate with them—things like attitude, body language, and word choice. But it goes even further to discuss the neurochemicals that drive these perceptions. Understanding all these different factors can help us approach conversations and communications with openness to promote superior outcomes.

Armed with the knowledge and skills you'll gain from reading this book, you'll be able to quickly identify when a conversation isn't going the way you intended and get things back on track.

Goals for This Book

This book is intended to:

- Present easy-to-recall acronyms to help you improve your conversation skills.
- Provide tips and techniques to help you overcome that "deer in the headlights" feeling that often occurs during difficult conversations.
- Offer direction and guidance for having critical conversations.
- Help you understand how various personality types match up with various traits and perceptions.
- Help you improve your communication by using empathetic language, body language, listening skills, and your own communication style.

- Teach you how to reduce your stress levels *before* a difficult conversation and help you make good decisions in the face of conflict to mitigate negative reactions.

How This Book Is Organized

Conducting a conversation is a little like driving a car. If you're not careful, you may find that people try to "run you off the road." For this reason, I structured the chapters in this book using a car metaphor. Each chapter is broken down into the following sections:

- **In the Driver's Seat:** This section introduces the main ideas in the chapter.
- **Your Road Map:** This section describes how you apply the main idea.
- **The Drive Home:** This section summarizes key points into bullets for easy review.

More on the Use of Acronyms

In addition to using a car metaphor to structure each chapter, this book also frequently uses a CAR acronym. CAR stands for:

- **C**onsideration
- **A**ction or a call to action
- **R**eturn on investment

You'll learn more about this concept starting in Chapter 1.

CAR is just one acronym used in this book. Another is BEST, which I consider the guiding principle for critical conversations. BEST stands for:

- **B**ody language
- **E**motional intelligence
- **S**cripting techniques
- **T**ips and techniques

Special Features

Throughout this book, you'll also find these special features:

- **Reflection boxes:** These challenge you to take a moment to consider how you can apply what you've learned.
- **Tip boxes:** These provide quick tips that you can apply to improve the effectiveness of your conversations.
- **Real World boxes:** These provide examples of research on effective communication techniques and relevant research articles.
- **Sidebars:** These provide important information that goes above and beyond the main text in the chapter.
- **Scripts:** Scripts for various types of common workplace conversations are provided throughout the book to give you examples of how to frame your conversations.

1

The Importance of Effective Communication in Healthcare

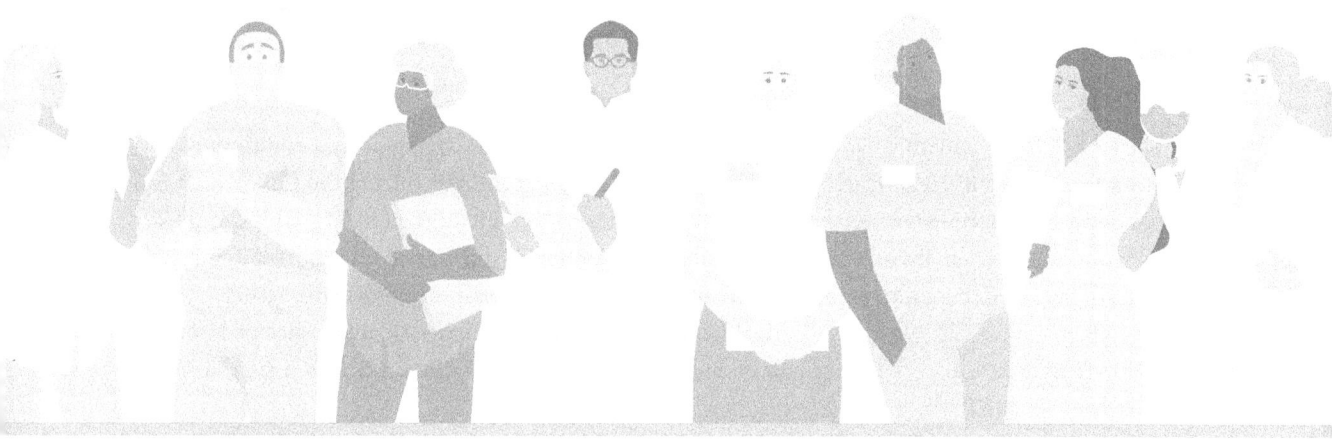

"Connection is the energy that exists between people when they feel seen, heard, and valued; when they can give and receive without judgment."
–Brené Brown, research professor and author

Dr. Brown's quote underscores the importance of connection in communication and how it requires sincerity, openness, empathy, and nonjudgmental listening. When we feel seen, heard, and valued in our interactions with others, we are more likely to feel connected and build meaningful relationships. Brené Brown's work underscores the role that vulnerability and authenticity play in nurturing connections and building trust with others.

With that in mind, I will ask you to breathe…with a short inhale and long exhale. I want to begin this chapter with an authentic and genuine *thank-you* for enduring a very sensitive and challenging pandemic. Although I'm unsure whether you are rolling your eyes while reading the words "thank you" or if you are smiling and interpreting it as an appreciation for all you and others have done during the last few years, I am still extending a very sincere thank-you that I hope is heard and valued.

Allow me to expound more on my dichotomy. Some of you may be thinking about yourself or someone you knew who experienced anything but a "thank-you" from healthcare leaders, organizations, or others by being furloughed, laid off, or placed in challenging and even unethical situations during COVID-19. The "thank-yous" we heard in the media were, at times, very undermining and even insulting. On the other hand, some of us experienced a thank-you with a sincere sense of pride and privilege—that we were able to help others and we were supported with proper resources, acknowledgements, and funds. Regardless of the acknowledgement you interpreted, I feel it is only appropriate to believe that no one will ever understand what you, I, we, or they experienced during the COVID-19 pandemic.

The COVID-19 pandemic has led to many personal, professional, spiritual, and emotional scars and triumphs. Healthcare staff who have been on the frontlines during the COVID-19 pandemic have faced enormous emotional and mental strain, including anxiety, stress, and burnout. Researchers found that more than half of healthcare staff surveyed reported symptoms of burnout, including emotional exhaustion and depersonalization (Nigam, 2023; Shanafelt et al., 2022). Additionally, healthcare staff working in high-risk areas, such as intensive care units, are at even higher risk of developing post-traumatic stress disorder symptoms (Kisely et al., 2020).

The impact of COVID-19 on healthcare staff worldwide was immense and brought to light how instrumental the critical role of effective communication was, and still is, in supporting anyone who works in or receives healthcare—that equates to *all of us*.

Connecting through communication is an important aspect of the human experience, as it allows us to form relationships with others and to feel a sense of belonging. It is through our communication styles that we share experiences and emotions with others and can receive support and understanding in return. Communication is the foundation of empathy, which helps us to see and experience the world from another person's perspective.

Hierarchy of Needs

Abraham Maslow's hierarchy of needs theory model (see Figure 1.1) exemplifies and reminds us of the connections between empathy and communication, as these concepts are pivotal to understanding human behavior and intrinsic and extrinsic motivation (Maslow, 1987).

Maslow's hierarchy of needs theory suggests that humans have a set of basic needs that must be met before they can reach their full potential. These needs include physiological needs such as food, water, and shelter, as well as safety needs, love and belonging needs, esteem needs, and self-actualization needs.

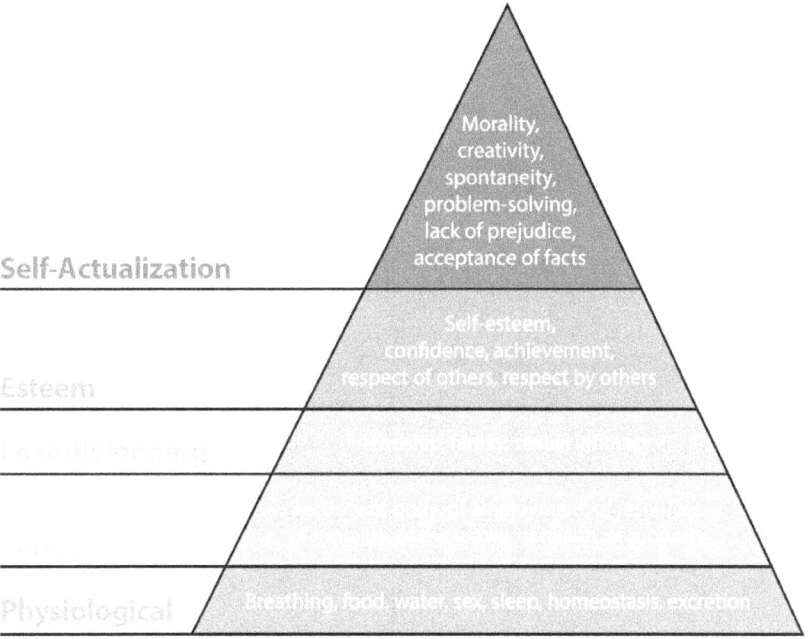

Figure 1.1 Maslow's hierarchy of needs.

Maslow's hierarchy of needs is often depicted as a pyramid with five levels, with the most basic needs at the bottom and the most advanced needs at the top. The first level is physiological needs, which includes the fundamental necessities of life such as food, water, shelter, air, and sleep. Without these needs being met, a person cannot progress to higher levels of the hierarchy.

The second level is safety needs, which includes the need for physical safety and security. This includes protection from harm, such as violence and disease, as well as a sense of predictability and stability in one's environment.

The third level is love and belonging needs, which involves the need for social connection and intimacy. This includes the need for friendships, family, and romantic relationships, as well as a sense of community and belonging.

The fourth level is esteem needs, which includes the need for self-esteem and recognition from others. This includes the need for respect, achievement, and recognition for one's accomplishments.

The fifth and final level is self-actualization, which involves reaching one's full potential and achieving personal fulfillment. This includes the need for creativity, autonomy, and the pursuit of personal growth and development.

Aligned with the concepts in Maslow's theory, Mary Kay Ash, the founder of Mary Kay Cosmetics in 1963, began her company as a small direct sales business. She sold skin care products and cosmetics through a network of independent beauty consultants. Today, Mary Kay Cosmetics is a global beauty brand, with operations in more than 40 countries worldwide.

She believed in empowering women to achieve their goals and to reach their full potential. Her leadership philosophy was based on the principles of recognizing, rewarding, and empowering her employees, and creating a positive and supportive work environment. She contributed to her company's success by sharing with her team, "Everyone has an invisible necklace around their neck that says, 'Make me feel important.' Always remember this when interacting with others." Essentially, Ash committed to focus on basic human needs—needs like love, belongingness, esteem, and even self-actualization—when communicating with others. She believed this was why her business was so successful. When you think about it, it's just common sense.

Still, as observed by Voltaire (BrainyQuote, n.d.), "Common sense is not so common." I believe this is because our human experiences are defined by our unique blend of interpretations, beliefs, feelings, values, culture, and morals. How can there be "common" sense when each person's sense of the world and of reality is so different? Add to that the role emotions play in our lives. Our emotions drive our thoughts, our thoughts drive our behaviors, and our behaviors drive our outcomes. If you've ever thought, "I'm just not in the mood for this today," then you understand the central role emotions play in our day-to-day interactions. Dealing with our own emotions is hard enough, let alone trying to deal with someone else's. It's not always easy to see that necklace!

I believe we can make common sense more common by focusing on basic human needs to improve the human experience. Case in point: If all healthcare begins and ends with the patient, why do we fall short in instilling behaviors and systems that center on patients? In fact, according to a recent Centers for Medicare & Medicaid Services Hospital Consumer Assessment of

Healthcare Providers and Systems (HCAHPS) survey, only 70% of patients would rate their hospital stay with the highest score (HCAHPS, 2024). For healthcare organizations, making a concerted effort not to just care for patients, but to care *about* them, just makes sense. After all, doing the right thing is always the right thing to do!

In the Driver's Seat: Finding Common Sense in Not-So-Common Conversations

Conceptually, *common sense* is centered on averages—what a typical response would be in an aggregate setting. A lack of common sense indicates that someone or something did not act in the average, standard, normative, or typical manner. Common sense is quite subjective because there are different perceptions of what is considered "common" to various people.

For example. there was a team of us working on a project to promote team engagement. One of our team members, Tony, was responsible for a specific task. Tony had been working on this task for several days, and during that time, he had come up with a plan to complete it. However, when he presented his plan to us, we did not understand it and had many questions about it.

To Tony, his plan seemed like common sense, but we just couldn't understand any part of it. Tony became frustrated and even shared that maybe we had the wrong group put together. After several days and upon a lot of reflection, Tony realized that he had not communicated his plan effectively to us, and that he needed to explain it in a different way to make it more understandable.

In this scenario, Tony assumed that his plan was common sense because he had been working on it for several days and had become familiar with it. However, we couldn't see it in the same way. This highlights the importance of effective communication and the need to listen, ask open-ended questions, and manage our emotions.

Let's look at another example. Have you ever been involved in a conversation in which everyone appears to agree on the matter at hand except you? I'm not talking about a small conversation during your lunch break. I'm talking about sitting in a large conference room, watching everyone else nod in agreement with the speaker, while you couldn't disagree more. This goes to show that even "majority rule" does not always reflect common sense—nor does it mean the majority is correct. Remember: Although averages can be informative, they do not provide a complete picture. To identify common sense, we must consider both the averages and variations of situations, as well as errors that can be perceived differently.

Let's consider this point on an even more granular level. Imagine a one-day post-op cardiac patient. His sternum has just been cut open. For him, moving his body at all—with the swan catheter, chest tube, IV lines, pain, etc.—is difficult, and practically impossible without help. Now imagine a dietary employee coming into the patient's room, leaving a liquid meal with all the wrapping on the juices intact on the table tray adjacent to the patient, saying to him, "Enjoy," and walking out.

I shared this scenario with a group of dietary employees and asked them to identify any errors made. The comments I received from the group indicated she had done nothing wrong. She delivered the correct food on time, moved the table close to the patient, and behaved cordially toward the patient. She did everything she should have done!

Then I shared the same scenario with a team of nurses. They were outraged. They asked how that patient was supposed to open the lids on the juices, let alone reach for the cup or open the straw based on the current state of the patient. They asked why dietary didn't open the juice for the patient, place a napkin on his lap, or even tell him they would let someone know (the nurse or the aide) that his food had arrived and that he needed assistance. "Dietary employees have no common sense!" they said.

When we talk about common sense, we need to examine the averages of how people look at things, the variations of how good care versus bad care can be perceived, and the understanding of what constitutes errors. Was this scenario a case of a knowledge deficit on the part of the dietary team in what the patient could or couldn't do? Or was it a case of, they'd better hurry up and deliver the food trays to all the patients so they don't receive poor service ratings? If someone does something that seems outside the bounds of common sense to you, consider why he might have done what he did. Unfortunately, small acts of kindness and thoughtfulness sometimes don't occur because some organizations have become so fixated on meeting metrics that they do not account for the things that can't be measured.

In this example, the problem was remedied by informing dietary team members of the limitations of patients and explaining that they should either ask family members (if available) if they would like to assist in feeding the patient or inform the patient that they would let the nurse know the tray is there and that the patient needs assistance.

Recognizing Differences in Interaction Styles

When people react to situations in a manner opposite from what you would do, it is easy to judge and make inferences. Instead, we need to identify and understand our behavioral differences. Researchers in the fields of social and industrial psychology offer insight into four personal or social styles (Bolton & Bolton, 2009; Merrill & Reid, 1981; Tracom Group, n.d.). This model, called the Social Styles Model (see Figure 1.2; Merrill & Reid, 1981; Tracom Group, n.d.), helps us improve communication and the quality of our relationships. It's important for me to explain that the Social Styles Model is not a comprehensive personality assessment or diagnostic tool. It's simply a framework for understanding varying behavioral styles that can be useful for communication and relationship-building purposes.

Understanding how each style interacts with others can help individuals tailor their communication approach to be more effective in different situations.

The four social styles are as follows:

- **Driving ("Get it done"):** People with this social style regulate their emotions in such a way that they may be perceived as aggressive and stoic. Drivers like to take control of situations, and they move quickly to get things done. Although they are known to be highly efficient, they are generally not sensitive to the needs of others. They typically do not consider others' feelings in their decision-making, nor do they take time to build strong relationships.
- **Amiable ("It's all about teamwork"):** People with this social style emphasize building and sustaining relationships. They tend to be agreeable and shy. Because cooperation is important to these folks, they tend to get caught up in everyone else's feelings and interactions rather than the task at hand.
- **Analytical ("Show me the facts"):** People with this social style like quantified content and thrive on factual data. They focus on logic and accuracy and stick to the facts. Although they prefer to work alone, they are still cooperative and approachable. Analytics like to take their time when making decisions so that all objective information is included and correct.
- **Expressive ("Commend and compliment"):** People with this social style are enthusiastic, attention-seeking, and alluring. They work to build continuous relationships with others and like to be recognized for their accomplishments. Expressive people use metaphors and move their bodies when speaking. Although others see them as artistic, they can appear frazzled, fragmented, or unsettled due to their excitement.

People with the expressive and amiable social styles have a humanistic interaction style, whereas people with driving and analytical social styles are more pragmatic and performance-driven.

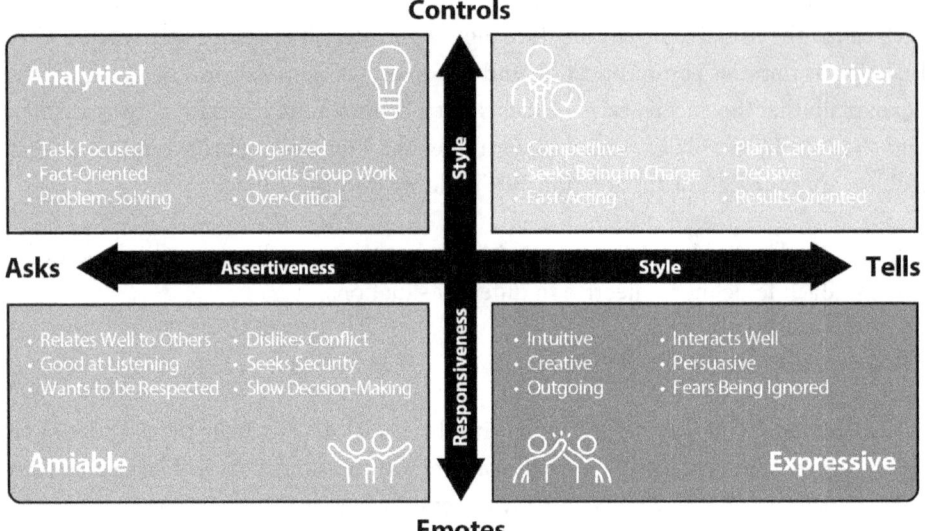

Figure 1.2 Social Styles Model.

Understanding Your Own Social Style and Others'

As you review the different social styles, you may have been wondering where you fall yourself, or are analyzing the people you live or work with. From a work perspective, you may notice some patterns in social styles across different departments or service lines. For example, people who work in information technology are likely to fall more into the analytical style, while managers may be more of the driver style. Remember that social style assessments are not definitive, and you may exhibit different social styles depending on the situation and context. But understanding other people's social styles can help you determine which position or role fits someone the most.

To determine your social style, you can take a social style assessment. There are many different social style assessments available, and some are more comprehensive and reliable than others.

Here are two examples:

1. DISC Assessment: The DISC assessment categorizes people into four social styles: Dominant, Influential, Steady, and Conscientious. The assessment measures how you behave in various situations and provides insight into your communication style, work preferences, and relationships.

2. Social Styles Model (as used as an example in this chapter): The Social Styles Model measures how you behave in various situations and provides insight into your communication style, decision-making, and leadership.

Understanding other people's social style can help you interact with others more effectively. Understanding how to flex to others social styles is beneficial for several reasons:

1. **Improved communication:** People with different social styles may have different communication preferences and tendencies. For example, an analytical person may prefer detailed information and facts, while an expressive person may prefer a more engaging and enthusiastic approach. Understanding someone's social style can help you tailor your communication to their preferences, which can lead to clearer and more effective communication.

2. **Better relationships:** When you understand someone's social style, you can adapt your behavior to better match their style. This can lead to a more positive and harmonious relationship, as you're able to communicate and interact with each other more effectively.

3. **More effective teamwork:** When working with others, it's important to understand their social style and work preferences. For example, an amiable person may prefer a collaborative and supportive work environment, while a driver may prefer a more fast-paced and goal-oriented approach. By understanding each other's social styles, you can work together more effectively and achieve better results.

4. **Increased empathy and understanding:** Understanding other people's social style can help you be more empathetic and understanding towards them. You may be better able to recognize their strengths and weaknesses and appreciate their unique perspective and contributions.

Adapting one's social style to align with the preferences of others can help to create more effective communication and build stronger relationships. Consider what style you identify the most with and try flexing to others' styles by using some of these tactics (see Figure 1.3):

1. **Analytical style:** Since analytical people tend to be logical, detail-oriented, and reserved, be prepared and organized. Provide clear and concise information and avoid making assumptions or generalizations. Allow time for them to process and analyze information before expecting a response, and be patient if they ask for additional information or clarification.

2. **Driver style:** Driver people tend to be assertive, decisive, and results-oriented. To interact effectively, be direct and to the point. Clearly communicate expectations and deadlines, and focus on outcomes and results. Be prepared to answer questions and provide justification for your ideas, and avoid getting bogged down in details or emotions.

3. **Amiable style:** Amiable people tend to be friendly, cooperative, and supportive. To interact effectively with amiable individuals, you'll want to build trust and rapport by listening actively and showing interest in their ideas and opinions. Avoid being confrontational or critical, and focus on finding common ground and building consensus.

4. **Expressive style:** Expressive people tend to be outgoing, enthusiastic, and spontaneous. To interact effectively with expressive individuals, it's important to be engaging and enthusiastic. Provide emotional support and connection, and focus on building a positive and energetic environment. Be prepared for changes and surprises, and avoid being overly critical or negative.

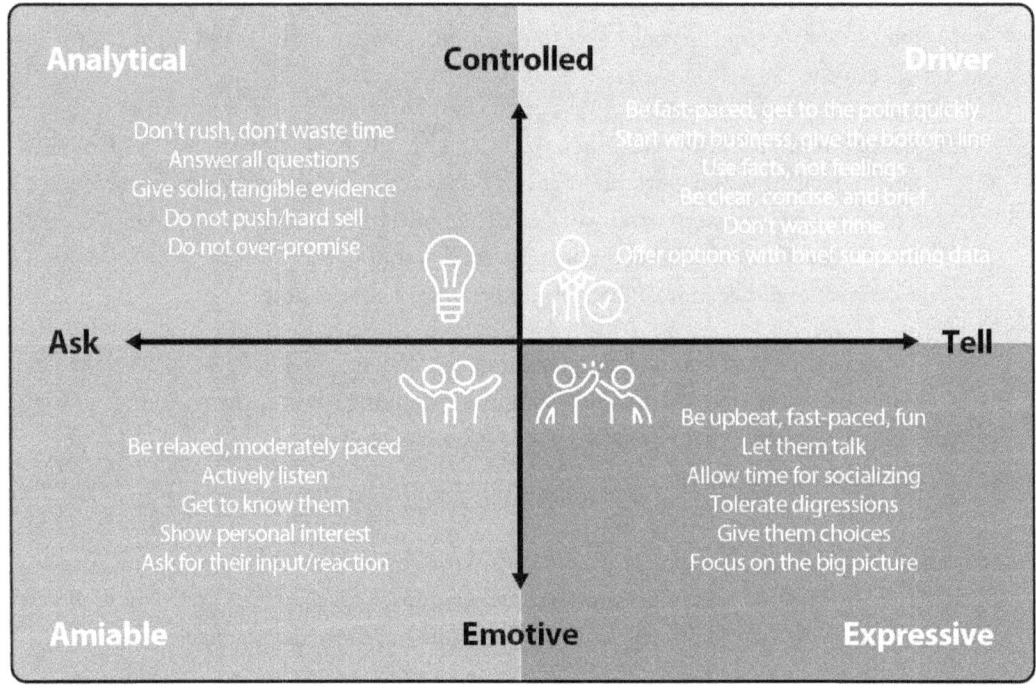

Figure 1.3 Flexing to style preferences.

Our awareness of these styles helps us to become more effective in how we communicate and interact with others. It's important to keep in mind that social style assessments are not definitive and should be used as a tool for self-awareness and personal growth. While your social style may be influenced by your personality, upbringing, and cultural background, it's possible to develop skills and behaviors that allow you to interact effectively with people of different social styles.

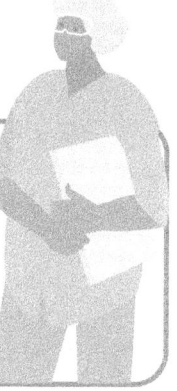

> ### Time to Reflect
>
> Everyone has a primary social style. Although these styles may overlap, we tend to have one that is more dominant. Take a moment to think about what your primary and secondary social styles are and how that might affect your communication with those who have differing styles.

The Benefits of Understanding the Social Styles in Healthcare

Consider how nurses with different social styles explain medication to patients. Again, note that these examples are simplified and generalized. In reality, individuals may exhibit a combination of different social styles, and it's important to adapt communication accordingly.

Analytical Style

Nurse: Good morning, Mr. Johnson. I wanted to discuss your new medication plan. Let's go through each medication one by one. This medication, prescribed by your doctor, is a beta-blocker. It works by slowing down your heart rate and reducing blood pressure. The dosage and timing are important, so I'll explain the recommended schedule in detail. Additionally, I have some informational pamphlets for you to review at your own pace. Feel free to ask any questions you may have.

In the given conversation, the nurse exhibits several characteristics of the analytical style. Let's break them down:

Thoroughness and attention to detail: The nurse expresses the intention to discuss the new medication plan with Mr. Johnson, indicating a desire to cover each medication comprehensively. This shows the nurse's commitment to providing a thorough understanding of the plan.

Systematic approach: The nurse suggests going through each medication one by one, indicating a structured and methodical approach to discussing the medications. This approach aligns with the analytical style's tendency to break down information into manageable components.

Focus on facts and information: The nurse provides specific information about the medication being a beta-blocker and its mechanism of action in slowing down the heart rate and reducing blood pressure. This emphasis on factual information demonstrates the nurse's inclination to provide accurate details for better comprehension.

Detail-oriented explanation: The nurse acknowledges the importance of dosage and timing and offers to explain the recommended schedule in detail. This focus on precise details reflects the analytical style's preference for ensuring accuracy and precision in conveying information.

Provision of resources: The nurse offers informational pamphlets for Mr. Johnson to review at his own pace. This demonstrates the nurse's recognition of the value of additional resources in supporting Mr. Johnson's understanding. Providing pamphlets aligns with the analytical style's inclination to provide supplementary information.

Encouragement of questions: The nurse invites Mr. Johnson to ask any questions he may have, indicating a willingness to address any concerns or uncertainties. This encourages a thorough exploration of the topic and highlights the analytical style's appreciation for precision through clarifications.

Overall, the nurse in this conversation displays several key characteristics of the analytical style, including thoroughness, attention to detail, a systematic approach, a focus on facts and information, detail-oriented explanation, provision of resources, and encouragement of questions. These characteristics contribute to the nurse's communication style and support the analytical style's preference for precision and accuracy in conveying information.

Driver Style

Nurse: Hi, Ms. Davis! I've reviewed your medication plan, and we need to make sure you're taking your medications on time. I'll create a schedule for you that outlines when each medication needs to be taken, including any special instructions like taking them with food. It's crucial to follow this plan precisely to maximize the effectiveness of the medications. I'll also set up reminders for you to ensure you don't miss any doses.

Here's a breakdown of the driver style characteristics highlighted in the conversation:

Direct and result-oriented: The nurse immediately addresses the importance of Ms. Davis taking her medications on time. This direct approach demonstrates the nurse's focus on achieving the desired outcome.

Efficient and task-driven: The nurse takes charge of the situation by offering to create a schedule for Ms. Davis that outlines the exact timing and any special instructions for each medication. This displays the nurse's goal of ensuring efficiency and adherence to the plan.

Emphasis on precision and effectiveness: The nurse emphasizes the crucial nature of precisely following the medication plan to maximize the effectiveness of the medications. This demonstrates the nurse's concern for achieving the desired results and highlights the importance of accuracy in carrying out the prescribed treatment.

Proactive approach: The nurse goes beyond simply providing instructions by offering to set up reminders for Ms. Davis. This proactive step shows the nurse's initiative in ensuring that Ms. Davis doesn't miss any doses, further highlighting the driver-like focus on efficiency and task completion.

In summary, the driver style in this paragraph is characterized by directness, efficiency, emphasis on precision and effectiveness, and a proactive approach to achieving the desired outcome of medication adherence.

Amiable Style

Nurse: Good afternoon, Mrs. Smith. How are you today? I wanted to talk about your medication plan. I understand that managing multiple medications can be overwhelming, so I'm here to help simplify things for you. We'll discuss each medication and its purpose, and I'll create a personalized schedule that fits your daily routine. I want to ensure you feel comfortable and confident about taking your medications. If you have any concerns or preferences, please let me know, and we'll work together to find the best solution for you.

In the given conversation, the nurse exhibits several characteristics of the amiable style. Let's break them down:

Warm and friendly approach: The nurse greets Mrs. Smith with a pleasant greeting and asks how she is doing, establishing a friendly and caring tone. This demonstrates the nurse's intention to create a positive and comfortable environment for the conversation.

Empathy and understanding: The nurse acknowledges the potential overwhelm of managing multiple medications and expresses empathy towards Mrs. Smith's situation. This understanding shows the nurse's compassionate approach and desire to address any concerns or difficulties Mrs. Smith may have.

Simplification and personalization: The nurse states the intention to simplify the medication plan for Mrs. Smith. By discussing each medication and its purpose and creating a personalized schedule that fits Mrs. Smith's daily routine, the nurse aims to alleviate any confusion and provide a customized approach to make medication management easier for her.

Focus on comfort and confidence: The nurse expresses the desire to ensure Mrs. Smith feels comfortable and confident about taking her medications. This focus on emotional well-being aligns with the amiable style's emphasis on creating a supportive and reassuring atmosphere for the individual.

Collaboration and open communication: The nurse encourages Mrs. Smith to voice any concerns or preferences she may have. By actively inviting her input and offering to work together, the nurse fosters a sense of collaboration and partnership in finding the best solution for Mrs. Smith's needs.

Overall, the nurse in this conversation displays several key characteristics of the amiable style, including a warm and friendly approach, empathy and understanding, simplification and personalization, focus on comfort and confidence, and collaboration and open communication. These characteristics contribute to the nurse's communication style and exemplify the amiable style's preference for building rapport, providing support, and ensuring the individual feels comfortable and heard during the conversation.

Expressive Style

Nurse: Hey there, Mr. Thompson! How's it going? Let's talk about your new medication plan. I'm excited because I believe it's going to make a big difference in managing your condition. These medications are powerful tools that can improve your health and overall well-being. I'll explain each medication's benefits and potential side effects, so you have a clear understanding. It's essential that you take them as prescribed, and I'll be here to support you every step of the way. Let's get started on this journey to better health.

In the given conversation, the nurse exhibits several characteristics of the expressive style. Let's break them down:

Enthusiastic and energetic tone: The nurse greets Mr. Thompson with an upbeat and friendly greeting, expressing excitement and enthusiasm. This sets a positive and engaging tone for the conversation.

Optimistic outlook: The nurse states that they believe the new medication plan will make a big difference in managing Mr. Thompson's condition. This positive outlook highlights the nurse's optimism and encouragement, aiming to inspire hope and motivation in Mr. Thompson.

Emotional language and connection: The nurse describes the medications as powerful tools that can improve Mr. Thompson's health and overall well-being. This use of emotional language aims to create a sense of connection and personal investment, emphasizing the potential positive impact on Mr. Thompson's life.

Clear explanation of benefits and potential side effects: The nurse assures Mr. Thompson that they will explain the benefits of each medication as well as potential side effects. This shows the nurse's commitment to providing comprehensive information, ensuring that Mr. Thompson has a clear understanding of both the benefits and the risks associated with the medications.

Support and presence: The nurse expresses their commitment to supporting Mr. Thompson every step of the way. This reassurance demonstrates the nurse's availability and willingness to provide assistance and guidance throughout Mr. Thompson's journey with the medication plan.

In healthcare, understanding the Social Styles Model can be valuable for effective communication and building strong relationships with patients and colleagues. Here are a few important points to know about the Social Styles Model in healthcare:

Communication styles: The Social Styles Model categorizes individuals into four main styles: analytical, driver, amiable, and expressive. Each style has distinct communication preferences, tendencies, and motivations. Recognizing these styles can help healthcare professionals tailor their communication approach to better connect with patients and colleagues.

Patient-centered care: Applying the Social Styles Model in healthcare enables providers to adapt their communication to the unique needs and preferences of individual patients. By understanding a patient's social style, healthcare professionals can adjust their approach to enhance patient engagement, trust, and satisfaction.

Team collaboration: The Social Styles Model is not limited to patient interactions but can also be useful in fostering effective collaboration among healthcare team members. By recognizing and respecting the different social styles of colleagues, healthcare professionals can improve teamwork, enhance cooperation, and reduce conflicts.

Nonverbal cues: Apart from verbal communication, understanding social styles can help healthcare professionals interpret and respond to nonverbal cues. Different styles may display distinct body language, tone of voice, and other nonverbal signals, which can provide insights into their needs, preferences, and comfort levels.

Flexibility and adaptability: It's important to note that individuals can exhibit a mix of social styles or may display different styles in different situations. Healthcare professionals should remain flexible and adaptable in their communication approach, considering the individual's unique characteristics rather than relying solely on stereotyping based on social styles.

Cultural sensitivity: Cultural backgrounds and personal experiences may influence individuals' social styles. It is crucial for healthcare professionals to be culturally sensitive and considerate of diverse perspectives and communication styles to ensure effective and respectful care.

By incorporating the Social Styles Model into healthcare practice, professionals can improve communication, enhance patient-centered care, strengthen teamwork, and foster positive relationships with patients and colleagues alike.

Taking the BEST Approach to Effective Conversations

Conversations can be considered effective when there is no error in the message as it relates to all participants. To decrease the chances of message errors, I like to use acronyms. Using the acronym BEST (see Figure 1.4) helps remind me of key components in conversations.

BEST stands for the following:

- **B**ody language
- **E**motional intelligence
- **S**cripting techniques
- **T**ips and tools

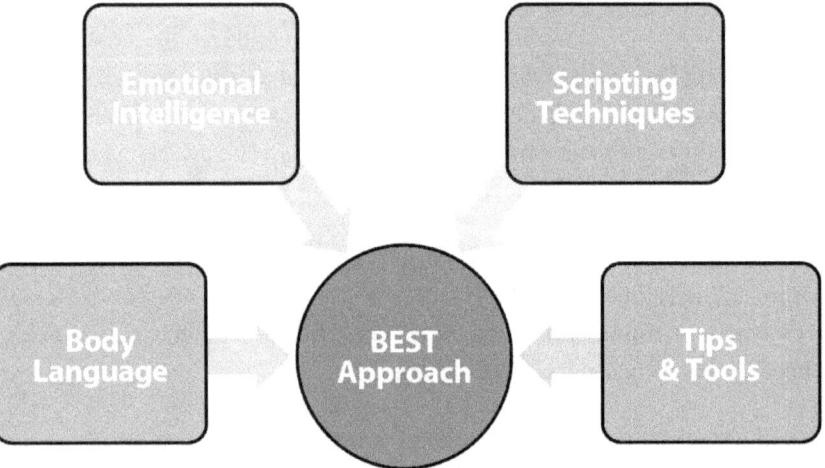

Figure 1.4   The BEST approach for effective patient and interprofessional conversations.

These are the key components that help drive effective conversations. If you can recall this acronym from memory, you can be confident that you're applying common-sense principles to even the most uncommon situations.

Think about a typical conversation at work. Before you start the conversation, you generally have some type of intention for it—small talk, factual, informative, or critical—even if you may not consciously be aware of it. This intention drives the flow of the conversation.

Although variations and deviations naturally occur in conversations, you can limit the extent of these variations and deviations—otherwise known as confusion—by applying the BEST acronym. For example, suppose the intent of a conversation with one of your patients is to assess her pain level. The patient says it is a 2 (with 5 being the worst pain), yet you notice the patient has increased respirations, is moaning, and appears very uncomfortable. If you apply the BEST acronym:

> **B** You'll notice that her *body language* is not congruent with her words.
>
> **E** Your *emotional intelligence* will remind you to be sensitive to how some patients may view pain medication because of fear of dependency, constipation, or shame, to name a few. (Chapter 3 discusses emotional intelligence in more detail.)
>
> **S** Using *scripting techniques*, such as recalling simple acronyms, will limit the variations and deviations in the conversation.
>
> **T** *Tips and tools* such as the use of open-ended questions help to keep communications a two-way conversation rather than a statement

So, rather than just accepting that your patient has minimal pain or saying to her, "Are you sure it's only a 2, Mrs. Davis?" ask her to tell you more about how she is feeling: "I hear you moaning and want to make sure you are resting comfortably. How can I help you be more comfortable?"

AIDET

Another common acronym that is considered a best practice by many healthcare organizations is AIDET. Studer (2003) introduced AIDET as a communication framework to decrease patient anxiety and increase patient compliance and outcomes. AIDET stands for:

- **A**cknowledge
- **I**ntroduce
- **D**uration

- **E**xplanation
- **T**hank you

AIDET can help ensure your conversation is comprehensive and clear, stays on the right course, and moves toward the correct conclusion. Of course, this is not to say that you follow the exact same sentence structure each time. For example, when acknowledging someone, you don't always have to say, "Hi, Mrs. Smith. It's nice to see you today." You'll have to customize the sentences relative to several variables, such as the person or situation. But using the framework in varying situations is helpful.

Consider the following script, which you could customize for a patient coming in for preadmission testing:

Acknowledge: "Hello, Mr. Franks. Could you please sign in? We can start getting you ready for your preadmission testing."

Introduce: "My name is Laura, and I've been a registered nurse here for about five years."

Duration: "You will most likely be here for about an hour. We will need to ask you some questions and assess you."

Explanation: "It's important that we ask some questions about your health, draw some blood, and take a chest X-ray. This information will help the doctor determine the best treatment plan for you. First, I need to ask you questions about your medical history. Next, I will take some blood. You will feel a pinch and pressure when I draw your blood. I will let you know when I'm about to do this if you'd like me to—some people would rather not know when the pinch is coming. You can let me know either way. Finally, you will have a chest X-ray. This is similar to having a picture taken. You won't feel any pain. What questions do you have for me?"

Thank you: "Thank you, Mr. Franks, for trusting me with your care. We have a great team here, and I'm happy to answer any other questions you may have."

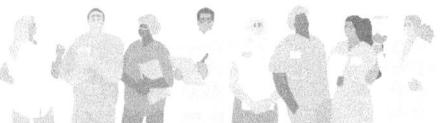

Body Language

Driver and van Aalst (2010) explain that when we interact with others, we continuously make and perceive gestures that either match what we are saying, are completely opposite to what we are saying, or both. All our nonverbal behaviors—the way we sit; the speed, inflection, and tone of our voice; how close we stand to another; how much eye contact we make; and so on—send strong messages that can either help or hinder our ability to effectively converse and affect our credibility.

Messages don't stop when we stop talking. Our bodies are still communicating whether we like it or not. Often, there is a vast dichotomy between what words we choose and what our bodies say. When faced with these mixed signals, the listener must decide whether to believe the verbal or the nonverbal message we are sending. Typically, the listener will choose to believe the nonverbal message because it is more likely to reflect our true feelings, thoughts, and intentions.

Here's a simple example: Have you ever asked someone, "Are you OK?" and received the answer, "Yes, I'm fine," even though the person's head and shoulders are slumped over, and he doesn't make eye contact? This simple example demonstrates how people may say one thing yet show another. (Chapter 2 expands on this idea.)

Consider Kevin, a new nurse manager of a 14-bed step-down unit, who called a staff meeting to share his action plan for improving patient experience. During the meeting, he noticed that many of the nurses nodded their heads vigorously in response to almost everything he said. He took this as a sign of success. As he reflected on the meeting afterward, he felt glad that he had added in a few facts to bolster his action plan, although it had lengthened the meeting by a few minutes.

After the meeting, only two of the 25 nurses chose to sign up for the "patient experience" committee he had outlined during the meeting. This confused Kevin because he had spoken at length about this great idea, and all the nurses had nodded their heads to agree with him as he spoke.

When he confronted the nurses later that afternoon, most said they didn't have time to sign up because they were late for another meeting. Kevin asked them to sign up by the end of the day. None of the nurses did. Why do you think this happened? Were the nurses really engaged? (Chapter 2 explores head nodding and other body language gestures in more detail.)

The Power of Body Language

Body language is very powerful. Even the most subtle, discreet body gestures can reveal tremendous amounts of information. Take, for instance, how different a conference call feels from sitting in an actual room with someone. The difference we perceive between these two environments is due to the vast amount of extra information we either gather or don't gather from body gestures. From the angle of our eyebrows to the direction of our feet, subtle body gestures can reveal a lot more than what is said.

- Body language can help you understand different personalities so you don't judge others.
- Body language conveys truth, even when words do not.
- Body language enhances listening and communication skills.
- Body language allows you to hear between the words spoken to understand what is being said.

- Understanding body language helps you identify your own body movements that hinder or foster success.

What's *really* powerful about body language is that we are not even cognizant we are giving more information than we may want to. Bottom line: Your emotions and behaviors are closely connected. As observed by American author John Maxwell (n.d.), "People hear your words, but they feel your attitude."

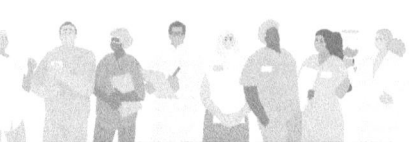

Emotional Intelligence (EI)

Goleman (2005) posited that our brain defaults to reacting and protecting us when faced with adversity. This can arise before we can rationally think things through. For example, suppose you are caring for a 66-year-old diabetic patient who won't stop yelling at you—and you have no idea what you did to upset her. If you're a person with low EI, you might immediately take this situation personally and yell back at the patient in a poor attempt to stop her from shouting. If you're a person who has high EI, you would calm yourself down, gain your composure, and then, using a soft, normal tone of voice, say something like, "How can I help you?" or, "I need you to speak slowly so I can better help you."

The REAL WORLD

Jiao et al. (2018) found that nurses with higher EI scores were associated with higher levels of patient-centered care. *Patient-centered care* is a healthcare approach that prioritizes the patient's needs and preferences, making it crucial for nurses to have the skills to provide this type of care effectively.

A systematic review conducted by Ko et al. (2020) found that higher EI in nurses was associated with better communication, empathy, and overall nurse-patient interaction.

Effective communication and empathy are critical components of providing quality care, and nurses with higher EI can better connect with their patients and provide care that meets their unique needs.

Nurses with higher EI scores are better equipped to provide patient-centered care, improve patient satisfaction, and provide a better overall care experience for their patients. Healthcare organizations should invest in EI training for nurses to improve patient outcomes and enhance the overall quality of care.

Time to Reflect

Here's an example story depicting an argument between an expressive nurse named Sarah and a driver nurse named Alex:

Sarah, an expressive nurse, bursts into the nursing station, visibly frustrated, and approaches Alex, a driver nurse who is known for being direct and results-oriented.

Sarah: Alex, I can't believe you didn't follow through with the patient's request for pain medication! It's crucial to address their needs promptly, and you completely disregarded their concerns!

Alex: Sarah, I understand your concern, but I had urgent tasks to complete, and I couldn't attend to the patient immediately. Prioritizing tasks is essential to keep everything on track.

As the argument escalates, tensions rise between Sarah and Alex. To resolve the conflict, here are some tips:

Active listening: Both Sarah and Alex should take a step back and actively listen to each other without interruption. This allows them to understand each other's perspectives and concerns.

Empathy and understanding: Sarah and Alex should try to empathize with each other's point of view. Sarah can acknowledge the importance of prioritizing tasks, while Alex can recognize the significance of promptly addressing patient needs.

Constructive communication: Encourage Sarah and Alex to express their thoughts and concerns in a respectful and calm manner. They should avoid personal attacks and focus on the topic at hand.

Seeking common ground: Identifying areas of agreement and shared goals can help Sarah and Alex find common ground. They can emphasize their shared commitment to patient care and the importance of effective communication within the team.

Compromise and collaboration: Encourage Sarah and Alex to explore potential solutions that address both the patient's needs and task priorities. They can work together to find a compromise or develop strategies that ensure patient care remains a priority without compromising other essential responsibilities.

Mediation or facilitation: If necessary, a neutral third party, such as a charge nurse or team leader, can mediate the conversation to facilitate a productive resolution. They can provide guidance, maintain a neutral standpoint, and help the nurses find a mutually agreeable solution.

In the end, resolving the argument requires open communication, understanding, and a willingness to find common ground. By actively listening, empathizing, and seeking compromise, Sarah and Alex can move forward, ensuring both patient care and task management are effectively addressed.

Our emotions can get the best of us unless we become aware of them and learn how to control them. We can't always avoid adversity, but we can change the way we react to it. Our behavior is cardinal to the way we communicate. Think about it: We hire staff based on their talent, and we fire them due to poor behavior. Sometimes, staff members are victims of their own emotions, especially when emotions are running high and self-preservation kicks into overdrive. This typically ends with a suboptimal outcome.

The REAL WORLD
IDENTIFYING EMOTIONAL INTELLIGENCE

High EI can play a crucial role in calming down an angry patient. Here's an example scenario demonstrating the impact of EI in such a situation:

In a busy emergency department, a patient named John arrives, visibly agitated and frustrated. He has been waiting for a considerable amount of time, and his impatience has escalated into anger. The nurse on duty, Sarah, recognizes the importance of addressing John's emotions and utilizes her high EI to de-escalate the situation.

Sarah approaches John calmly, maintaining a friendly and composed demeanor.

Sarah: "Good afternoon, John. I apologize for the wait. I understand you're frustrated, and I want to help. Can you please tell me what's been going on?"

John, still visibly upset: "I've been waiting for hours, and nobody seems to care. This is ridiculous!"

Sarah acknowledges John's feelings and validates his concerns.

Sarah: "I completely understand why you're frustrated, John. Waiting can be really frustrating, especially when you're not feeling well. I'm sorry for the inconvenience caused. Let's see how we can address your concerns and get you the care you need."

Sarah's empathetic response and acknowledgment of John's emotions demonstrate her high EI. She shows genuine concern for his well-being and takes the time to listen to his frustrations.

Sarah: "While I check on the status of your care, I want to assure you that we value your time and well-being. I'll do my best to provide you with an update as soon as possible. In the meantime, is there anything I can do to make you more comfortable? Would you like some water or a magazine to read?"

Sarah's proactive offer to address John's immediate needs helps redirect his focus and provides him with a sense of control in the situation.

John, starting to calm down: "I appreciate that. Some water would be great."

Sarah retrieves a glass of water for John, using the opportunity to continue the conversation.

Sarah: "Thank you for your patience, John. I've spoken with the medical team, and they are working diligently to ensure you receive the care you need. I'll keep you updated on the progress. If there's anything else you need or any questions you have, please don't hesitate to let me know."

Sarah's continuous communication and transparency help establish trust and provide reassurance to John. By keeping him informed, she reduces his uncertainty and gives him a sense of being heard and valued.

As time passes, John's anger subsides, and he begins to feel more at ease. Sarah's high EI, demonstrated through empathy, active listening, validation, and proactive support, has effectively calmed down the initially angry patient.

By understanding and addressing the patient's emotions with empathy and patience, healthcare professionals like Sarah can de-escalate tense situations, restore trust, and create a more positive patient experience. High EI enables healthcare providers to navigate challenging interactions, promote effective communication, and ultimately improve patient outcomes.

Scripting Techniques

Scripting is a set of messages, phrases, or sentences that you can, without much thought, weave into conversations to organize the flow of the conversation. Scripting and other similar techniques enable nurses to deliver thoughtful and appropriate responses in an authentic way.

The TELL Acronym

The TELL framework for critical conversations is a structure that can be used to guide and navigate difficult or sensitive discussions. TELL stands for:

T - Time and place to talk: Choose an appropriate time and place for the conversation where both parties can have privacy, minimal interruptions, and sufficient time to discuss the matter thoroughly.

E - Explain and explore perspectives: Begin the conversation by exploring each person's perspective, feelings, and concerns. Encourage open and honest communication, actively listen to the other person's viewpoint, and seek to understand their position.

L - Listen to their perspective: Practice active listening and demonstrate empathy towards the other person's emotions and experiences. Validate their feelings and show understanding, even if you may disagree with their viewpoint. Avoid making assumptions or jumping to conclusions during the conversation. Focus on gathering information and understanding the complete picture before drawing conclusions.

L – Leverage shared values and lead the conversation forward: Be clear in expectations moving forward; the goal is to come to a mutually agreeable solution.

The TELL framework outlined here is a generalized approach to facilitate productive and respectful communication during difficult discussions.

Nurses can develop formats for scripts and for various situations. These scripts might consist of a single sentence, or they might contain the wording of an entire conversation. For example, Script 1.1 illustrates a conversation you might have with a colleague who isn't pulling her workload or weight. Script 1.2 is a more one-sided conversation you might have with a "difficult" patient. Tips and tools include active listening, displaying empathy, and asking open-ended questions.

When using an acronym or script, I can't stress enough how important it is to convey your message with authenticity. There is nothing worse than listening to some prescriptive jargon that has no real meaning or value. When used properly, scripting techniques can help deliver a consistent, meaningful, and comprehensive message. This is especially important in healthcare settings, where the error rate should be zero. When used improperly, acronyms and scripts can sound inappropriate or robotic.

Using open-ended questions is another way to incorporate scripting into conversations. An *open-ended question* is one that unobtrusively compels a person to volunteer more information (see Script 1.2 for examples). Using open-ended questions can help us ensure that what we said was actually heard. For example, the following three questions ask the same basic question, but each elicits a different response:

- Do you have any other questions for me?
- You don't have any other questions for me, do you?
- What questions do you have for me?

> People talk at roughly 200–250 words per minute (WPM) but can listen at 300–500 WPM (Douglass & Douglass, 1993). Don't underestimate what others hear or understand when you talk!

The first question is a closed question, requiring a simple yes/no response. The second question is a leading question; in other words, it leads the person to answer the question in a certain way. The third question is an open-ended question. This type of question takes out any bias or conclusions because it neither confirms nor denies what was perceived and understood. Using words like *what*, *why*, and *how* is an excellent way to ensure your questions are open-ended.

Scripting and the Service Industry

The service industry became enamored with scripting many years ago. Think about the service you receive at franchises such as Chick-fil-A or Starbucks. Almost every customer-service opportunity ends with a staff member saying "My pleasure" after being thanked by a customer.

The hotel industry is another example. Many front-desk and concierge staff use open-ended scripts. Consider the difference between asking, "Did you have a pleasant stay with us?" versus, "How was your stay with us?" The former is more likely to elicit a yes/no response from the guest, while the latter may elicit more feedback, such as, "It was a great stay! The view was awesome," or, "I've had better. I waited over an hour for room-service delivery." This feedback, whether positive or negative, is valuable information to identify wins and reveal opportunities.

Integrating Teach-Back Into Your Conversations

Weaving scripting and teach-back methods into conversations enables nurses to maintain a level of flexibility in dialogue. In *teach-back,* asking the patient to "teach back" what was said ensures information is understood. This is very effective even for the purposes of the HCAHPS survey. This survey is sent by the government after select patients are discharged from a hospital and asks core questions about a patient's hospital experience. Some of the domains include communication with doctors and nurses, the quality of information given at discharge, transitions of care, room cleanliness, medication understanding, and noise level in patient rooms. Let's look at a sample HCAHPS question:

How often did hospital staff describe possible side effects in a way you could understand?

When hospital staff use the teach-back method with patients, it helps patients recall and identify possible side effects. This leads patients to answering "always," or top box (the highest rating on the survey), for that question. Teach-back is also universally accepted as a best practice to overcome health illiteracy. *Health illiteracy* is an inability to understand basic health information and services needed to make appropriate health decisions and follow instructions for treatment (Schillinger et al., 2003). Thirty-six percent of Americans are below a basic health literacy level. Remember: Conversations are only as good as one's ability to communicate value and meaningfulness to others. In other words, if we don't articulate the importance of what we are trying to say to others, the information will go in one of their ears and out the other.

SCRIPT 1.1

What to say when…

A NURSE COLLEAGUE IS NOT FULFILLING THEIR RESPONSIBILITIES.

T
Time and place to talk

Choose an appropriate time and place to have a conversation with your supervisor. Find a quiet and private setting where you can discuss the issue without interruptions.

Example: Hi [colleague's name], do you have a moment? I wanted to discuss something important regarding our work responsibilities. Can we find a time to talk privately?

E
Explain and explore perspectives

Clearly, empathetically, and objectively explain the specific instances or observations where you have noticed that your colleague is not fulfilling their responsibilities. Use concrete examples to support your concerns, ensuring that your feedback is specific and constructive.

Example: I've noticed that there have been several occasions recently where tasks assigned to you, such as completing patient assessments or documenting vital signs, have been left incomplete or delayed. For instance, yesterday, I had to cover for you during the morning shift because several patient assessments were not done.

L
Listen to their perspective

Give your colleague an opportunity to share their perspective and express any challenges they may be facing. Actively listen without interruption and seek to understand their side of the story.

Example: I'd like to hear your perspective on this matter. Are there any specific challenges or difficulties you've been facing that have affected your ability to fulfill your responsibilities? It's important for us to have open communication and support each other.

L
Leverage shared values and lead the conversation forward

Remind your colleague of the shared goals you both have as healthcare professionals. Emphasize the importance of teamwork and the impact of each person's contributions on patient care outcomes.

Example: As a healthcare team, our ultimate goal is to provide the best possible care for our patients. By working together and fulfilling our responsibilities, we can ensure their well-being. Let's find ways to support each other in achieving these goals.

Example: To ensure that patient care responsibilities are consistently met, let's discuss strategies that can help you stay on track with your tasks. We could explore options like better time management techniques, delegation of certain tasks, or additional support from our team.

By utilizing the TELL framework, you can approach the conversation in a respectful and constructive manner, addressing the issue of your colleague not fulfilling their responsibilities while maintaining a focus on finding solutions that benefit both patients and the healthcare team.

SCRIPT 1.2

What to say when…
YOU GREET AN UPSET PATIENT.

T
Time and place to talk

Choose an appropriate time and place to approach the upset patient. Find a quiet and private area where you can have a conversation without distractions or interruptions.

Example: Excuse me, [patient's name], do you have a moment? I would like to talk to you in a more private area where we can discuss your concerns.

E
Explain and explore perspectives

Explain to the patient that you'd like to understand the situation more, or simply show empathy toward the patient's emotions and demonstrate that you understand their distress. Use active listening skills to let the patient express their concerns and feelings.

Example: I can see that you're upset, and I want you to know that I'm here to listen and help. Please tell me what's on your mind so that I can better understand your situation.

L
Listen to their perspective

Give the patient your full attention and actively listen to their concerns. Allow them to express their thoughts and feelings without interruption. Validate their emotions and reassure them that their concerns are important.

Example: I hear your frustration, and I understand that you're feeling upset. It's completely understandable given the situation you're in. I want to assure you that we're here to address your concerns and find a resolution.

L
Leverage shared values and lead the conversation forward

Ask the patient what they think may be a plausible solution or address their concerns. Offer reassurance that you will do everything possible to assist them and ensure their needs are met.

Example: Let's work together to find a solution. I'll do my best to address your concerns and provide the support you need. Is there anything specific you would like me to consider or any questions you have?

Here's an example: Suppose on the morning of surgery you ask an 80-year-old pre-op patient if he ate anything since midnight. He says, "No." You then ask him to share with you (teach) what he did that morning. He explains he woke up and had his normal coffee and just a bite of a cookie. He states that he "didn't eat anything"; he "just had a small bite." In other words, the patient perceived "didn't eat anything" to mean he hadn't consumed a full meal. You tell him that the surgery will need to be canceled because he had food. The patient replies that if the nurse who called him the night before had explained he couldn't even have a small bite of something, he wouldn't have had it. You explain about the risk of aspiration, and the patient replies that if they had explained this in detail to him the night before, he wouldn't have even had the coffee! All this is to say that if you hadn't asked him to "teach" or tell you the events of his morning, this pre-op no-no would have gone undiscovered. One of the best ways to ensure what you say is understood and perceived correctly is to have a person teach it back to you.

You must take control of the conversation when you do not understand someone or something or if you get the impression the person you're talking to isn't in tune with what you're saying. Recognize variances and deviations in what is being said versus what *isn't* being said by decoding body language, managing your emotions, and using acronyms and teach-back strategies. Do not always settle for yes/no responses when eliciting feedback. The next section discusses how you can pull all these tools together and use them as a road map to ensure your conversations are most effective.

The REAL WORLD
USING SCRIPTING TO IMPROVE PATIENT EXPERIENCE SCORES

Guimond-Lacroix et al. (2021) conducted a systematic review of literature to explore the effectiveness of scripting in improving patient experience scores in healthcare settings. The aim was to ensure that patients receive consistent and clear information and to promote patient-centered communication.

The authors reviewed 15 studies published between 2015 and 2020 that examined the use of scripting in various healthcare settings, including emergency departments, primary care, and outpatient clinics. They found that overall, scripting was associated with improvements in patient experience scores, particularly in domains such as communication, empathy, and patient satisfaction.

Your Road Map: Guiding Principles for Effective Communication

You can break down the process of communication into a simple three-step process, using the CAR acronym (which contains the BEST approach within it):

- **C**onsideration
- **A**ction or call to action
- **R**eturn on investment (ROI)

This acronym is your road map (no pun intended) to clearer, more focused, and more effective conversations. The CAR acronym can even be used when you're involved in an emotionally charged or controversial conversation.

Let's map out (pun intended) the CAR acronym so you can see how the BEST approach is embedded.

Consideration

The *C* in CAR means to *consider* the Five Rights of Communication Safety. These are as follows:

- **Right person:** You are speaking with the right person.
- **Right place:** You are having a discussion in the right place.
- **Right time:** It is the right time for the discussion.
- **Right emotions:** Your emotions are rightly in check (EI and body language).
- **Right ROI:** You have the right ROI, or intent.

Just as medication errors are frequently the result of a failure to check the Five Rights of Medication Safety, which you may recall from nursing school, communication errors are often the result of failing to check the Five Rights of Communication Safety. You can remember the Five Rights of Communication Safety with the CAR acronym.

Action or Call to Action

The next part of CAR is the *A*, which stands for *action* or *call to action*. This refers to the desired outcome for the conversation. Think of this as a backward approach to having a conversation. First you determine what response you hope or expect to receive from the listener.

In other words, you ask yourself, is the intent of the conversation to give directives, to coach, to complete a task, to seek more information, or to clarify something? With this outcome in mind, you think about what action you need to take to get the response you want.

The action or call to action is the engine of the conversation. It describes the organization of your thoughts throughout the conversation and the actual deliverable of the conversation.

Return on Investment

The *R* in CAR stands for the return on investment (ROI). This measures the effectiveness of your conversation. A high ROI means the investment gain or conversation outcome compares favorably to the investment cost—which, in the context of conversations, is typically how much time you took to get the desired result.

You can also consider the ROI to be high if you learned what worked or what didn't work in your approach. In this case the return is that you will be able to build on what you learned to get you the results you want. Evaluating your ROI is beneficial because it enables you to create a toolbox of communication strategies that will help you get the results you want when you need them the most.

CAR Example

Suppose the provider told your patient that he can be discharged this morning. It's now almost noon, and the patient—who is dressed and ready to go, and whose family is waiting patiently (although their patience is wearing thin)—is still waiting to be discharged because the provider hasn't entered the discharge order yet. You feel you should contact the provider and ask to have the discharge order entered. Sounds easy, right? Well, not so much if, for example, you know this provider doesn't like to be told what to do, or if they've just stepped off the unit, or what have you. So, what's the best way to proceed?

First you *consider* the Five Rights of Communication Safety:

- **Is the practitioner really the right person to speak with?** In other words, could the nurse practitioner write the order?
- **Is this the right place to discuss the situation?** The conversation should be held in a private room, not in another patient's room.
- **Is this the right time to discuss the situation?** If the provider is in the midst of running a code or even conducting interdisciplinary rounds, it might be best to wait another five minutes until the provider is done.

- **Are the right emotions in check?** If the provider is known to take direction poorly or to lash out when asked to do something, be prepared to approach them in a nonthreatening manner. Saying "Mr. Gonzales has been waiting a very long time and is getting angry at you since you have failed to put in *yet* another discharge order on time" can sound harsh and undermining. A better approach might be something like, "Just a friendly reminder to put in the discharge order for Mr. Gonzales. I want to make sure we are respectful of his time since he and his family have been patiently waiting for the order."

- **Do you have the right ROI or intent?** In this case, yes. You are advocating for the patient's time and overall patient bed flow.

Next you identify the action or call to action—in this case to prompt the provider (or nurse practitioner) to immediately enter the discharge order so you can properly discharge this patient. The ROI is that the provider respects your request, and Mr. Gonzales is sent on his way.

The Drive Home

Let's drive home the key points in this chapter:

- Common sense is subjective because different people perceive different things to be "common."
- A popular model used to improve interpersonal communications is the Social Styles Model.
- Each of the four social styles in the Social Styles Model has its own strengths in certain situations and offers opportunities when working with others.
- The BEST approach incorporates all the core components of an effective conversation, including body language, EI, scripting techniques, and tips and tools.
- A conversation is only as effective as our ability to clearly communicate its intent and purpose.
- The message our body language reveals can be completely opposite of the words we say. This can help or hinder conversation and even affect our credibility.
- EI reminds us that we can't always avoid adversity, but we can change the way we react to it.
- When seeking informative responses from people, we need to ask open-ended questions—that is, questions that start with what, why, and how.

- The CAR acronym is an overarching framework that includes the BEST approach. CAR stands for:
    - **C**onsideration: Consider the Five Rights of Communication Safety.
    - **A**ction or call to action: This is the foundation of the conversation—how you will respectfully articulate what you're seeking from the listener.
    - **R**eturn on investment (ROI): A high ROI indicates the conversation was successful and compares favorably to the amount of time you took to get the desired results.

References

Bolton, R., & Bolton, D. G. (2009). *People styles at work . . . and beyond: Making bad relationships good and good relationships better.* AMACOM.

BrainyQuote. (n.d.). *Voltaire quotes.* https://www.brainyquote.com/authors/voltaire-quotes

Douglass, M. E., & Douglass, D. N. (1993). *Manage your time, your work, yourself.* AMACOM.

Driver, J., & van Aalst, M. (2010). *You say more than you think: A 7-day plan for using the new body language to get what you want.* Crown Publishers.

Goleman, D. (2005). *Emotional intelligence: Why it can matter more than IQ.* Random House.

Guimond-Lacroix, A., Blais, R., Pomey, M. P., & Leclerc, B. S. (2021). Developing and testing a scripted communication intervention for nurses in primary care to improve patient experience. *Journal of Nursing Scholarship, 53*(1), 97–106.

Hospital Consumer Assessment of Healthcare Providers and Systems. (2024). *HCAHPS survey.* https://www.hcahpsonline.org

Jiao, H., Shi, Y., Li, D., Xu, X., & Zhang, H. (2018). Emotional intelligence and patient-centered care: A study of resident physicians. *Journal of Healthcare Management, 63*(2), 113–126.

Kisely, S., Warren, N., McMahon, L., Dalais, C., Henry, I., & Siskind, D. (2020). Occurrence, prevention, and management of the psychological effects of emerging virus outbreaks on healthcare workers: Rapid review and meta-analysis. *BMJ, 369.*

Ko, E., Kim, S. J., & Kim, M. S. (2020). The impact of nurses' emotional intelligence and communication satisfaction on their organizational commitment. *Journal of Clinical Nursing, 29*(19–20), 3711–3721. https://doi.org/10.3389/fpsyg.2023.1125465

Maslow, A. H. (1987). *Motivation and personality* (3rd ed.). Longman.

Maxwell, J. (n.d.). *30 inspirational John C. Maxwell quotes on leadership.* http://smartandrelentless.com/30-inspirational-john-c-maxwell-quotes-leadership/

Merrill, D. W., & Reid, R. H. (1981). *Personal styles and effective performance.* CRC Press.

Nigam, J. A. S., Barker, R. M., Cunningham, T. R., Swanson, N. G., & Chosewood, L. C. (2023). Vital signs: Health worker-perceived working conditions and symptoms of poor mental health–Quality of worklife survey, United States, 2018–2022. *Morbidity and Mortality Weekly Report, 72*(44), 1197–1205. https://doi.org/10.15585/mmwr.mm7244e1

Schillinger, D., Piette, J., Grumbach, K., Wang, F., Wilson, C., Daher, C., Leong-Gratz, K., Castro, C., & Bindman, A. B. (2003). Closing the loop: Physician communication with diabetic patients who have low health literacy. *Archives of Internal Medicine, 163*(1), 83–90. https://doi.org/10.1001/archinte.163.1.83

Shanafelt, T. D., West, C. P., Dyrbye, L. N., Trockel, M., Tutty, M., Wang, H., Carlasare, L. E., & Sinsky, C. (2022). Changes in burnout and satisfaction with work-life integration in physicians during the first 2 years of the COVID-19 pandemic. *Mayo Clinic Proceedings, 97*(12), 2248–2258. doi: 10.1016/j.mayocp.2022.09.002

Studer, Q. (2003). *Hardwiring excellence: Purpose, worthwhile work, making a difference.* Fire Starter Publishing.

Tracom Group. (n.d.). *The social style model.* https://tracom.com/social-style-training/model

2
Body Language Exposed

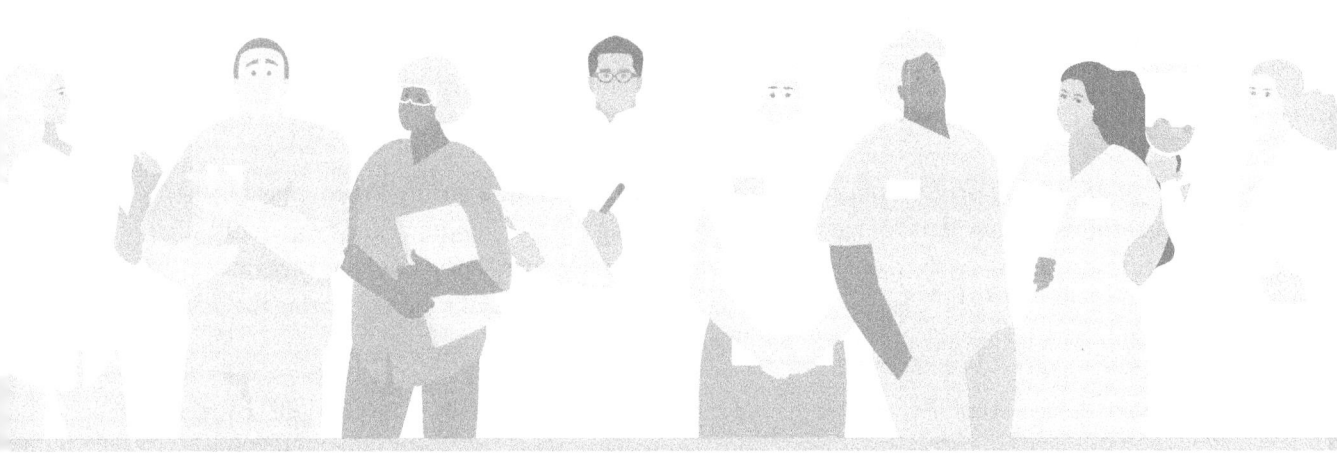

*"The most important thing in communication
is hearing what isn't said."*
–Peter F. Drucker

At a previous job, several directors and I were asked to attend a meeting with one of our newest senior directors, whom I'll call Mary. Mary was an extremely charming and charismatic leader with stellar business acumen and financial experience. Mary was also well educated, with more than 20 years of experience in healthcare executive management.

Before the meeting, Mary requested that each of us bring a few high-priority departmental issues to discuss. We were told that, based on these discussions, Mary would pick the top issues, which she would then prioritize in her new leadership role.

At the meeting, Mary gave a warm introduction, asked us to introduce ourselves, and then proceeded to solicit information about our departmental issues. While my colleagues and I took turns sharing our issues, I watched how Mary's body language changed based on some of the words she heard. Some of the many topics discussed included revenue cycle, charge entry, lack of resources, staffing issues, quality improvement, relative value units, value-based purchasing, and meaningful use dollars.

It wasn't just Mary's facial expression that I homed in on, but the position of her upper body (as we sat around the boardroom table), whether she was writing with her pen or just dangling it from her hand, how often she cupped her chin with her hand, and the direction of her eyes. For example, when my colleagues spoke of a lack of specific resources, I noted Mary feverishly writing on her pad, occasionally nodding, and cupping her chin with her hand. When colleagues spoke passionately about staff performance management issues, Mary looked up to the right and down to the left, sitting back in her chair.

I was one of the last of the directors to speak. I discussed clinical quality-improvement issues. As I spoke, I noted Mary looking to the right, smiling a lot, and nodding quite vigorously. After a brief discussion, as she had done with my colleagues, Mary said she would be very supportive in my endeavors. At the end of the meeting, Mary genuinely thanked us for sharing the information with her, and the meeting concluded on a positive note.

I have learned over the years that many people know just what to say to be politically correct, but most people aren't as experienced with—or even cognizant of—what their body language is saying. When you are adept in assessing body language, you can get a better sense of what someone is thinking, even if the person isn't speaking. Mary's body language revealed to me what she may have perceived listening to each of our topics.

Shortly after the meeting was adjourned, I quietly mentioned to one of my colleagues that I thought the issues I shared didn't make Mary's top-priority list. I also said I would be surprised if any of the staffing issues would be on the list, although 90% of us mentioned lack of staffing as an issue. He looked quite puzzled and asked me how I came to that conclusion. He reiterated how much Mary nodded and smiled to me as I spoke. He thought she appeared very engaged, especially because Mary pointed out to the group just how important my department was to the organization. I agreed with my colleague that what she said was supportive, but I also explained to him that I found a disconnect in her words and her body language. My colleague once again reassured me that Mary reacted no differently to me than she did to anyone else. He went on to say I was reading way too much into the situation and should be more optimistic.

So, who was right—my colleague or me? The email Mary sent shortly after the meeting confirmed that I was right. None of my issues made her top-priority list, nor did anyone's staffing issues. Meaningful-use dollars made the top-priority list, as well as a focus on revenue-cycle improvements. Can you guess why these issues made her top-priority list? If you said her priorities were fiscally related, not clinically related, you were right.

In the Driver's Seat: Understanding and Interpreting Body Language

In this chapter, I share common and not-so-common body-language tips and tidbits that can help you interpret what people are saying beyond the words they use. You can also apply this knowledge to improve your nonverbal communication strategies so that your own words and body language are congruent.

Between 50% and 80% of communication is nonverbal (Mehrabian, 1972, 1980). It is so important that we not only listen to others but also "hear" what their bodies say. Body language is a two-way street. Your body language can reveal to others feelings you are suppressing, and other people's body language can reveal their suppressed feelings toward you.

A considerable amount of information can be interpreted through body language. When you meet someone for the first time, you interpret information about the person even before words are exchanged. It takes only a few seconds to make a first impression. According to Mehrabian (1980), body language guides 55% of that impression, 38% comes from tone of voice, and the remaining 7% from your actual words.

The most obvious forms of body language are conveyed by our faces, eyes, and hands. Some less obvious forms of body language include the following:

- What we look at while talking or listening
- Our facial expressions, including the positioning of our mouths and eyebrows

> Although the interpretations of certain gestures may seem obvious to you as you read them in this book, things aren't always so clear in real life—especially if your attention is focused elsewhere due to difficult emotional circumstances (Businessballs, n.d.; Driver & van Aalst, 2010).

- Our body position
- The open space we leave between others when conversing (this is known as *proxemics*; what makes this interesting is how our body positions change during conversations)
- How and when we touch ourselves and others during conversations
- How our bodies touch tangible objects, such as pens, cigarettes, glasses, and clothing
- How fast we breathe and even how much we perspire

The following sections describe how our eyes, mouth, head, arms, hands, handshake, legs, feet, and personal space communicate our feelings to others. As you review each of these areas, note that there are no absolute interpretations for body gestures, merely suggested interpretations. To effectively interpret body language, all gestures need to be assessed as a whole. As Aristotle (Goodreads, n.d.) stated, "The whole is greater than the sum of its parts."

Body Language Traits Based on Social Style

Social psychology researchers introduced the four social styles discussed in Chapter 1. Each of these four styles is associated with certain types of body language (Bolton & Bolton, 2009; Merrill & Reid, 1981). For example:

- People with a driving social style make lots of direct eye contact and keep the space between them and the person with whom they are speaking very close. This positions them to stay in control of the conversation. People with this social style also use their hands and fingers in conversations to put emphasis on their key talking points.
- People with an expressive social style make intermittent eye contact and periodically touch others while speaking to emphasize their points. They are more likely to raise their voices when speaking and to talk quickly so they can keep up with all the thoughts racing through their mind. People with this social style are very visual and animated. They tend to use metaphors and their hands to articulate ideas and suggestions.
- People with an amiable social style maintain an appropriate amount of eye contact with others. They tend to stay at a distance or lean back when speaking to others because they are shy. They are soft-spoken and move at a slow pace.
- People with an analytical social style use eye contact intermittently, making more eye contact when driving a point and less when deliberating about something. Their bodies often appear rigid, and they tend to keep space between themselves and the listener.

Sources: Merrill & Reid (1981); Tracom Group (1991)

Eyes

We are naturally adept at gathering information just by looking at or into the eyes of others. Eye contact can be good, bad, or just plain awkward, depending on the context.

We know almost immediately when we make eye contact with someone else, even when we are a significant distance from them and can't see their eyes in detail. We can also determine when someone is staring awkwardly at us or taking a clandestine peek. We often make inferences about others just from how they use their eyes (Businessballs, n.d.; Driver & van Aalst, 2010). See Table 2.1 for a list of eye gestures and their meanings.

Table 2.1 Possible Meanings of Eye Gestures

GESTURE	POSSIBLE INFERENCE(S)	RATIONALE
Viewing right Viewing right and down Viewing right and up	Visualizing, creating, fabricating, guessing, lying, storytelling	Looking right typically denotes creativity or some sort of exaggeration. This could be as harmless as spinning a story for a child or attempting to embellish facts. Or it could mean telling an outright lie.
		Looking down and to the right indicates the person is accessing her feelings. This could be a perfectly genuine response, but the true genuineness depends on the context and the person.
		When accessing the right hemisphere of our brain, we look up and to the right. Therefore, this gesture often relates to imagination, creativity, or lying. This can be a warning sign that someone is lying if she is supposed to be recalling and stating facts.
Viewing left Viewing left and down Viewing left and up	Recalling, remembering, retrieving facts, truthfulness, self-talk, rationalizing	When recalling facts from memory, we use the left hemisphere of our brain. When someone looks to the left it typically indicates that she is telling the truth.
		Looking down and to the left may indicate the person is carrying on an inner conversation or strategizing how she might attempt to redirect the conversation.
		Looking up and to the left is a reassuring sign if the person is supposed to be recalling and stating facts.

continues

Table 2.1 Possible Meanings of Eye Gestures (cont.)

GESTURE	POSSIBLE INFERENCE(S)	RATIONALE
Direct eye contact while speaking	Honesty, faked honesty	Direct eye contact is generally regarded as a sign of honesty and truthfulness. However, practiced liars know this and will try to fake others out by using this technique.
Direct eye contact while listening	Attentiveness, interest, attraction	When a person's eyes are directed at the speaker's eyes, this indicates the person is focused, interested, and paying attention. This is normally a sign of attraction.
Widening of the eyes	Interest, appeal, invitation	When people are interested in something, their pupils dilate. Although eyes that are widened with eyebrows raised can signify shock or surprise, they can also represent an opening and welcoming expression.
Rubbing eye or eyes	Disbelief, upset, tiredness	Rubbing both eyes, or even only one eye, can indicate disbelief, as if someone is checking their vision. This gesture can also signal someone is upset and may indicate crying is imminent. Finally, it can mean tiredness from lack of sleep or due to boredom.
Rolling of eyes	Frustration	An upward roll of the eyes signals frustration or annoyance.
Blinking frequently	Excitement, pressure	The normal eye-blink rate ranges between six and 20 times per minute. Excessive blinking is a sign of excitement or pressure.
Blinking infrequently	Various	Infrequent blinking can mean different things, such as boredom or intense concentration.
Eyebrow raising	Greeting, recognition, acknowledgment	Quickly raising the eyebrows is a common signal of greeting and acknowledgment. A more elaborate eyebrow flash, where eyebrows are raised for a longer time, may indicate fear or surprise.
Winking	Friendly acknowledgment, complicity (e.g., in the case of a joke or a shared secret)	A wink is commonly a flirtatious or intimate signal, directed from one person to another. A wink can signal a shared joke or secret, hence its power.

Source: Adapted/paraphrased with permission from Businessballs.com (n.d.).

As you may have noticed, several eye gestures may reveal that a person is lying.

How to Tell if Someone Isn't Being Honest With You

A useful acronym to help you identify these and other body gestures that suggest someone may be lying is 2BROKE. This acronym stands for:

- **2B:** Blinking and brow movements
- **R:** Right-sided eye movements (if the person is right-handed)
- **O:** Opposite mirroring
- **K:** Knuckles clenched
- **E:** Edgy (fidgety, nose rubbing, staring, no silence)

> **Key takeaway:** By keeping the "2BROKE" acronym in mind, you can enhance your ability to spot potential dishonesty, allowing you to make more informed decisions and maintain healthier relationships.

Be aware that it is very hard for someone who is being dishonest to resist speaking if you go silent. The person wants you to believe his lies, so he often scrambles to fill the silence. Script 2.1 shows you how best to deal with a colleague's dishonest behavior.

Mouth

The mouth is associated with multiple body-language signals because it can be touched or concealed by a person's hands, fingers, or other objects. We associate the mouth not only with speech but also, as you may recall from your study of Sigmund Freud during your nursing-school days, with infant feeding, which further connects it psychologically with feelings of security, affection, love, and sex. Although more obvious mouth gestures, such as smiling, are huge components of facial body language, the extent of a person's smile has different meanings. For example, real smiles are symmetrical and produce wrinkles around the eyes and mouth, while forced smiles don't. With a forced smile, only the mouth crease changes (Businessballs, n.d.; Driver & van Aalst, 2010). See Table 2.2 for a list of various mouth gestures and their meanings.

SCRIPT 2.1

What to say when…

YOU ARE CONFRONTING A COLLEAGUE'S DISHONEST BEHAVIOR.

T

Time and place to talk

Choose an appropriate time and place for the conversation. Find a private setting where you can have a focused discussion without distractions.

Example: Coworker

> Shane, telling our boss you had to leave the meeting early because of an issue with one of your patients is wrong—we both know that. If our boss asks me about this, he will easily catch me in a lie since the chart doesn't reflect your story.

E

Explain and explore perspectives

Clearly and objectively explain the specific instances or observations where you have noticed your colleague's dishonest behavior. Use concrete examples and facts to support your concerns.

Example: Guilt Trip

> Look, you know this interview is extremely important to me. I wouldn't ask you to do this unless it was important.

> I want to help you out. I understand you needed to leave the mandatory meeting to take a phone call about your upcoming job interview at Hospital ABC. I really hope you get the job. I think you'll probably be a lot happier there. In the meantime, I need this job, and I'm afraid our manager will take action against me when she finds out I'm covering for you.

L
Listen to their perspective

Give your colleague an opportunity to share their perspective and provide any explanation for their behavior. Practice active listening and seek to understand their side of the story.

Example: Continuing Guilt Trip

> *Just say it is something about the family—something we don't document. Say anything like that. Please?*

> *I can tell our manager I knew you had to step out, but I'm not comfortable telling her it was a patient-care issue. I will just tell her I'm not really sure what was going on—since I really don't know what happened on your call.*

L
Leverage shared values and lead the conversation forward

Remind your colleague of the shared values and expectations within the workplace. Emphasize the importance of integrity, honesty, and the impact their actions have on patient care and the overall reputation of the team.

Example: Thankful

> *That is fine. I really owe you one. Thanks again!*

> *I can do this, this one time for you. I don't like to be placed in this difficult situation. Please don't ask me to cover again. It's not because I don't want to help you; it's because I need this job. I appreciate your understanding my situation, too.*

Table 2.2 Possible Meanings of Mouth Gestures

GESTURE	POSSIBLE INFERENCE(S)	RATIONALE
Forced smiling	Fake smile	A fake smile may indicate disapproval or feeling forced into doing something the person does not want to do.
Smiling without showing teeth	Withholding feelings or comments	The person may have a secret he is trying not to disclose.
Smiling with lips closed and edges of mouth pulled back toward ears	Fake smile	This is the epitome of a fake smile. The jaw is dropped low, and the mouth appears long.
Smiling with the head tilted sideways and down but the eyes looking up	Playfulness, flirting, teasing	This head position partially obscures the person's face and smile. This is an effective way to draw in someone's attention.
Bottom lip salient	Upset, empathy	A salient bottom lip—that is, a lip that is pushed forward—signals imminent crying and upset. It may also be an overt attempt to seek sympathy or kind treatment. Sometimes people push out their bottom lip in a playful manner or even in an authentically empathetic way.
Laughing naturally	Relaxation	Natural laughter is a sign of relaxation. It can cause the person to change the position of his upper body or even his whole body.
Laughing unnaturally	Nervousness, cooperation	Unnatural laughter is often a signal of nervousness or stress. It can also be a subtle signal to try to get others to cooperate.
Biting lip	Stress, anxiousness	Biting the lip can be caused by stress or anxiousness.
Chewing on an object	Self-comforting, flirting	Nibbling on an object—for example, a pen—can suggest oral pleasure. (Think about the message you're sending to colleagues or patients when you chew on the end of a pen or pencil during a conversation with them!)

GESTURE	POSSIBLE INFERENCE(S)	RATIONALE
Pursing lips	Thoughtfulness, impatience	This often happens when people are trying to hold words in their mouth or stop themselves from talking over someone. This can also indicate anxiousness or impatience at not being able to speak at that time.
Poking tongue	Disapproval, rejection	This gesture is similar to the reaction people have when they taste something gross. This is even more obvious when the person's nose wrinkles and eyes squint.

Source: Adapted/paraphrased with permission from Businessballs.com (n.d.).

Head

Because our brains are located inside our heads, the head guides our general body direction. Our heads are used in a lot of directional (approving and disapproving) self-protection (defensive or offensive) body language. A simple turn or tilt of the head has various meanings, providing significant information about what's *not* being said. Our heads, especially when our hands interact with them, can be dynamic in communicating all sorts of messages, both consciously and unconsciously (Businessballs, n.d.; Driver & van Aalst, 2010). See Table 2.3 for a list of various head gestures and their meanings.

Table 2.3 Possible Meanings of Head Gestures

GESTURE	POSSIBLE INFERENCE(S)	RATIONALE
Nodding head up and down	Understanding, agreement	Nodding our heads shows we agree with or understand what the other person is saying.
Nodding head up and down slowly	Attentive listening (could also be fake)	Although this gesture could authentically reveal that the person is listening, it can also be a faked signal. If the person is making eye contact with you, then it suggests she is listening.

continues

Table 2.3 Possible Meanings of Head Gestures (cont.)

GESTURE	POSSIBLE INFERENCE(S)	RATIONALE
Nodding head up and down fast	Hurry up, impatience	Nodding your head fast indicates you've heard enough and you're ready to move on to something else.
Holding head up	Neutrality, alertness	This can show attentive listening and/or that the listener is not biased one way or the other about what you are saying.
Holding head up high	Superiority, fearlessness, arrogance	Keeping your head raised displays confidence. It can also be valuable for demanding respect and showing authority.
Tilting head to one side	Nonthreatening, submissive, thoughtfulness	Head tilts suggest we may be considering a different view of the other person or subject. Head tilting also exposes our neck, which is a sign of trust.
Tilting head downward	Criticism	Tilting our head downward is a sign of criticism or disapproval.
Shaking head side to side	Disagreement	This gesture can indicate disagreement or reveal feelings of disbelief.
Pronounced head shaking	Strong disagreement	A more pronounced shaking of the head can show how strongly we feel about someone or something.
Placing head down	Negative, embarrassment, shame	We use head-down gestures when we are responding to criticism. This gesture can indicate failure or feeling embarrassed or shamed.
Holding chin up	Pride, defiance, confidence	Holding your chin up exposes your neck and is a signal of trust, strength, confidence, resilience, pride, etc. It also lifts the sternum, which improves airflow, expands the chest, and widens the shoulders. This can make a person's stance appear superior. An exposed neck is a sign of confidence.

Source: Adapted/paraphrased with permission from Businessballs.com (n.d.).

Arms

Our arms can reveal a lot about our mood and feelings. For example, crossing our arms may mean we are defensive. However, it could also mean we are bored or trying to self-regulate because we feel insecure or upset. (Remember: No gesture has one single, absolute meaning!) In contrast, we open our arms wide to indicate we are open or accepting of others. See Table 2.4 for a list of various arm gestures and their common meanings.

Table 2.4 Possible Meanings of Arm Gestures

GESTURE	POSSIBLE INFERENCE(S)	RATIONALE
Crossing arms	Defensiveness, reluctance, physically cold	We often cross our arms when we feel threatened by others. We also cross our arms when we are physically cold or when we are bored.
Crossing arms with tightened fists	Hostility, defensiveness	Keeping our fists tight with our arms crossed in front of our chest may indicate that we feel stubborn or aggressive, or that we lack empathy. Watch out: When you see this gesture, it means defenses are raised high!
Gripping own upper arms	Insecurity	When we feel afraid or unsafe, we tend to cross our arms with our hands holding the opposite arm. This is also known as self-hugging.

Source: Adapted/paraphrased with permission from Businessballs.com (n.d.).

Hands

Our hands contain more nerve connections to the brain than almost any other part of our body. Indeed, Driver and van Aalst (2010) observe that our hands reveal almost as many signals as our faces do. For this reason, our hands often express what we are thinking or feeling. We use our hands a lot in both conscious and unconscious gesturing (Businessballs, n.d.). For example, communicating with our hands can demonstrate:

- **Importance:** Examples include pointing, poking, slowing-down, and speeding-up motions.
- **Illustration:** These types of gestures include gestures that imitate drawing, mimicking actions, signals such as the thumbs up or OK sign, or motions that attempt to illustrate the size of something.
- **Salutations:** Waving hello or goodbye are examples of salutations.

Studying hand body language provides a lot of information. See Table 2.5 for a list of various hand gestures and their meanings.

Table 2.5 Possible Meanings of Hand Gestures

GESTURE	POSSIBLE INFERENCE(S)	RATIONALE
Placing open palm(s) up	Passive, trustworthy, appealing	This gesture often indicates openness. It can also mean, "I don't know." Be careful, however: This gesture can easily be faked to look innocent.
Facing palm(s) toward the listener with fingers pointing up	Defensive, stop gesture	With this gesture, fingers are rigid, indicating an authoritative instruction to stop whatever is going on.
Placing palm(s) down	Authority, strength, dominance, calm-down gesture	Moving one's lower arm across the body with the palm down is generally a sign of defiance or disagreement. It could also mean the person is asking the listener to calm down.
Placing palm(s) up and moving up and down as if weighing something	Seeking an answer	This indicates that one is figuratively holding an issue, as if measuring its weight.
Placing hand(s) on heart (left side of chest)	Seeking to be believed	We use this gesture to convince the listener to believe us—whether we are being truthful or not.
Pointing finger at a person	Aggression, threat, emphasis	Pointing at a person is very confrontational and dictatorial. This indicates a lack of social awareness or self-control, not to mention arrogance, on the part of the finger pointer.
Pointing finger with a wink	Acknowledgment, confirmation	Winking one's eye at someone while pointing a finger at them typically means one is acknowledging something. This can be a signal of positive appreciation, as if to say, "You got it."
Pointing finger in the air	Emphasis	When we point a finger in the air, we are generally trying to add emphasis to something.
Wagging finger side to side	Warning, refusal	This is like saying "no" or asking the listener to stop.

GESTURE	POSSIBLE INFERENCE(S)	RATIONALE
Wagging finger up and down	Admonishment, emphasis	People sometimes finger-wag up and down, as if they have an imaginary yo-yo in their hand, to keep the listener in rhythm with what they are saying or to emphasize their point.
Making hand-chop gesture	Emphasis	We often use a hand-chop motion to place a strong emphasis on a point we are trying to make or to indicate that we are attempting to end a discussion with power.
Clenching fist(s)	Resistance, aggression, determination	Clenching one's fist can indicate different feelings, such as defensiveness or negativity, depending on context. A clenched fist is an attempt to prepare oneself for battle.
Steepling fingers pointing up	Thoughtfulness, looking for or explaining connections, engagement	In this gesture, the tip of each finger and thumb touches the corresponding digit of the other hand and points upward like a church steeple (hence its name). People who perceive themselves as being intellectual often do this because it conveys elevated thinking.
Steepling fingers pointing forward	Thoughtfulness, defensive barrier	This is similar to the preceding gesture, but with the fingers pointing forward. It acts as a defensive barrier between people.
Clenching or interweaving fingers	Frustration, negativity, anxiousness	This gesture signals that emotions are high. This is especially true when hands turn red or bluish from the tight grasp.
Touching the index finger and thumb at the tips and pointing remaining fingers up	Satisfaction	This is the "OK" signal.
Pointing thumb(s) up	Positive approval, agreement	A thumbs-up means "approved." It's a positive gesture. However, it can also be done facetiously.
Pointing thumb(s) down	Disapproval, failure	A thumbs-down means "not approved" or indicates poor performance.
Clenching thumb(s) inside fist(s)	Self-comforting, frustration, insecurity	This gesture tends to indicate the person is self-comforting, but it may also mean they're holding something back.

continues

Table 2.5 Possible Meanings of Hand Gestures (cont.)

GESTURE	POSSIBLE INFERENCE(S)	RATIONALE
Holding hand horizontally and rocking it from side to side	Undecided, in the balance	We may see this when a decision or outcome is difficult to predict or control, as it is viewed as going one way or another.
Rubbing hands together	Anticipation	This shows positive expectations and is often seen as a favorable response to rewards, activities, meals, or outcomes.
Touching or scratching the nose while speaking	Lying, exaggeration	Although people often scratch their nose when recounting an event or incident (or if they just have an itch), it can also indicate lying.
Pinching or rubbing the nose while listening	Thoughtfulness, suppressing comment	This gesture indicates one is holding back information or thinking hard to recall something.
Pinching bridge of nose	Negative evaluation	We often pinch the bridge of our noses as a negative response to something. This is typically done while holding a long, single blink.
Clamping hands over ears	Rejection, resistance to something	This signifies an unwillingness to hear what is being said or viewed.
Tugging ear	Indecision, self-comforting	Ear tugging can indicate one is pondering or is indecisive. However, touching our bodies in various ways often signals we are seeking comfort. Ear tugging is one such comforting gesture.
Clasping hands on head	Calamity	Clasping one's hands on one's head is like putting on a protective helmet against a problem or a response to a panicked "oh, no!" thought.
Stroking chin	Thoughtfulness	This gesture is like the one made by a man using his thumb and index finger to stroke his beard. It indicates that someone is giving something thoughtful consideration.
Supporting chin or side of face	Evaluation, tiredness, boredom	When we support our heads or chins with our hands, we are assessing or evaluating next actions, options, or reactions to something or someone.

GESTURE	POSSIBLE INFERENCE(S)	RATIONALE
Resting chin on thumb with index finger pointing up against face	Evaluation	This gesture is similar to the previous one but is a more reliable signal of evaluation.
Scratching neck	Doubt, disbelief	When we hide our necks in any way, we are showing feelings of distrust.
Clasping wrist with hand	Frustration	Clasping the opposite wrist with our hand—either behind our back or in front of our pelvic region—can be a signal of frustration, as if we are holding ourselves back.
Covering pelvic region with clasped hands	Nervousness, defensiveness, protectiveness	This is another type of protective gesture. We also use this gesture when we are trying to appear formal or ready (but still feeling nervous deep down; Driver & van Aalst, 2010).
Holding hands together behind body	Confidence, authority	This confident stance is often assumed by military personnel, teachers, police officers, and so on.
Running hands through hair	Flirting, exasperation	Running one's hands through one's hair is commonly associated with flirting. It can also indicate we are feeling exasperation.
Placing hand(s) on hip(s) ("Superman" pose)	Confidence, readiness, availability	This stance emphasizes our presence and shows our readiness for action.
Placing hands in pockets	Disinterest, boredom, confidence	When our thumbs are tucked inside our pockets, we are typically not ready for action. However, when our thumbs are held outside our pockets, we show confidence.
Holding a drink, pen, or something else across the body while seated	Nervousness	This defensive gesture indicates nervousness or discomfort.
Removing glasses	Desire to speak	People who wear glasses may remove them to show others they want to speak. This gesture attracts attention to the face.

Source: Adapted/paraphrased with permission from Businessballs.com (n.d.).

Handshake

A firm handshake demonstrates confidence and poise. A firm handshake with a smile is commonly used to establish a trusting relationship. Handshakes that are obnoxiously firm, however, show a lack of respect (Businessballs, n.d.; Driver & van Aalst, 2010).

Although many people believe confident people give firm handshakes, I know many confident people who offer timid handshakes. I often see this when men gently shake a woman's hand out of respect for their femininity. Many of my female colleagues—even ones who are pit bulls in the boardroom—tell me they shake other women's hands with extreme gentleness as a sign of respect. The bottom line: Do not judge someone simply based on the strength of their handshake. Instead, look at where their palms are facing during the handshake. This will tell you so much more. See Table 2.6 for a list of various types of handshakes and their meanings.

Mutual Handshake

In Figure 2.1 notice how the palms are parallel. This signifies a mutually respectful relationship.

Dominant/Submissive Handshake

In Figure 2.2 notice how one palm is facing down and the other is facing up. The palm that is facing down signifies dominance, and the palm facing up shows submissiveness.

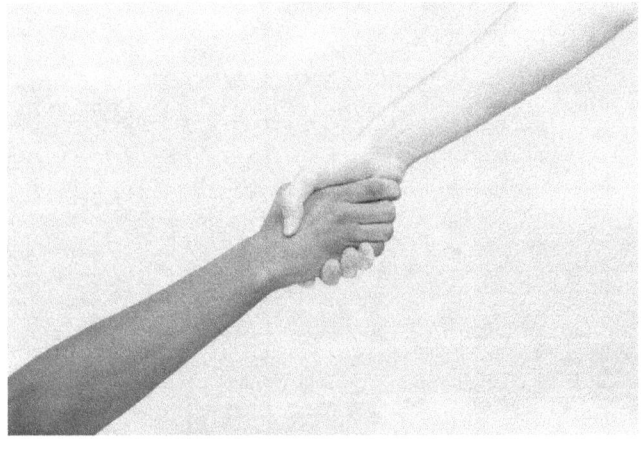

Figure 2.1 Mutual handshake.

> ### Time to Reflect
>
> If you wanted to make a good impression on someone, where would you aim your palm to face? If you guessed parallel, you guessed correctly because you want to show you are trustworthy and confident (not submissive or dominant).

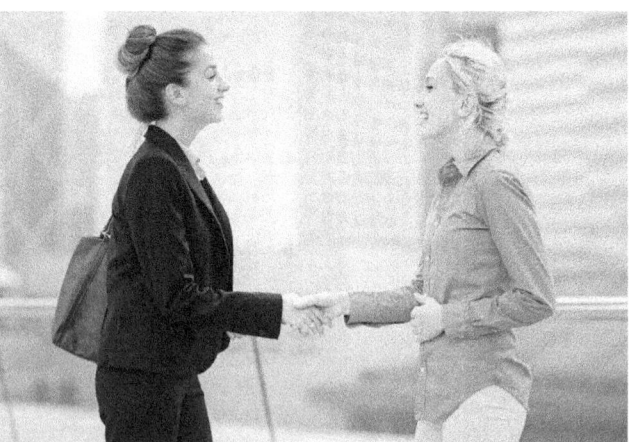

Figure 2.2 Dominant/submissive handshake.

Table 2.6 Possible Meanings of Types of Handshakes

GESTURE	POSSIBLE INFERENCE(S)	RATIONALE
Shaking hands with the palm down	Dominance	If you shake someone's hand firmly with your palm down and above theirs, you're expressing dominance. In other words, you have the "upper hand."
Shaking hands with the palm up	Submission, accommodating	This occurs when your hand is placed in a submissive palm-up position by the other person's dominant hand. This is typically considered a weak handshake.
Shaking hands with the palm vertical	Nonthreatening, relaxed	This is typical of most handshakes, when no one seeks to dominate or submit to the other person.
Giving a pumping handshake	Enthusiasm	This type of vigorous pumping handshake tends to indicate energy and enthusiasm.
Giving a weak handshake	Various	Avoid the common view that a weak handshake is the sign of a weak or submissive person. Weak handshakes may in fact be due to various aspects of personality, mood, and so on.
Giving a firm handshake	Outward confidence	A firm handshake is a sign of outward confidence, which could indicate a strong person or could mask deceit.
Shaking hands while clasping the recipient's arm or covering the joined hands with the other hand	Seeking control, care	A handshake accompanied by the left hand clasping the other person's arm or covering the handshake can indicate a desire to control something. It can also mean the person is adding an extra gesture of caring.

Source: Adapted/paraphrased with permission from Businessballs.com (n.d.).

Legs and Feet

The direction in which our legs and feet are pointing provides some insight to our feelings and moods. Note, however, that when sitting for extended periods, people naturally change their body position. Therefore, you should not gauge others by the way they are sitting at any one time. Instead, assess a person's posture as a whole throughout the entire conversation. See Table 2.7 for a list of various leg and feet gestures and their meanings.

> Leg gestures tend to be supported by corresponding arm signals, so review both body parts. For example, a person may cross her arms and legs for comfort, but that posture may also indicate detachment or disinterest (Businessballs, n.d.; Driver & van Aalst, 2010).

Table 2.7 Possible Meanings of Gestures With the Legs and Feet

GESTURE	POSSIBLE INFERENCE(S)	RATIONALE
Leg direction	Interest, attentiveness (according to direction)	The direction in which our feet or knees are pointing indicates where our interest is. The opposite is also true: If our legs or knees are pointing away from something or someone, it may indicate that we consider that thing or person uninteresting or threatening.
Sitting with uncrossed legs (men)	Openness	Men who sit with their legs uncrossed are generally expressing an open attitude.
Sitting with open legs spread wide (men)	Arrogance, combativeness, sexual posturing	This posture can be considered aggressive or arrogant because it takes up space and makes the person appear larger. However, this position could also just be physically comfortable for larger men.
Sitting with legs together in parallel (women)	Properness	This posture is common in women who have been taught to follow traditional rules of etiquette. To many, this is the proper posture for a lady.
Sitting with crossed legs (general)	Caution, disinterest	Crossed legs tend to indicate a degree of caution or disinterest. This can be for various reasons, ranging from feeling threatened to mild insecurity. However, many women naturally sit like this, so the key here is to pay attention to the direction of the knee. Typically, the knee will point toward what the person views as most interesting. This could be another person or even the door.
Sitting with legs crossed in figure-4 position	Independent, stubborn	In the figure-4 position, the ankle or calf of one leg rests on the knee of the supporting leg, creating a shape like the number 4. This posture, which exposes the pelvic area and usually causes the upper body to lean back, conveys confidence.
Sitting with legs crossed in figure-4 position with hand(s) clamped around knee	Resistant, stubborn	Clamping one's hand(s) around the knee of the top leg is a locked, defensive, or resistant gesture.
Sitting with ankles locked	Defensiveness	Clasping one's ankles tightly around each other is a defensive gesture. It may also indicate the person is uptight or nervous.

GESTURE	POSSIBLE INFERENCE(S)	RATIONALE
Sitting with legs interwoven (women)	Insecurity, sexual posing	In this posture, one leg is twined or wrapped around the other. This can be a sign of insecurity or indicate a need for protection. Note, however, that some women may sit like this to appear long and lean.
Standing with legs wide	Shield or protect	This stance acts as a foundation to shield or protect and gives the appearance of a broad body frame. Placing one's hands on one's hips enhances this impression, as in a prominent Superman pose. (Refer to Table 2.5.)
Standing at attention	Respectful	In this position—called "at attention" in the military—the person stands upright, with his legs straight, together, and parallel; his shoulders back; and his arms by their sides. This stance is considered to be respectful.
Standing with legs crossed (scissor stance)	Insecurity, submission, engagement	This position, in which the person's legs are crossed but their arms are not, can indicate a submissive or steadfast agreement to stand. It can also show the person is engaged. Scissor legs result in a shapely silhouette, which is why many celebrities and models pose like this for the paparazzi.
Standing with foot forward	Directed toward dominant group member	Although this is a small gesture, it can reveal a lot. People typically direct their feet toward the person they consider to be the most dominant member of a group. If one foot is facing out, however, it may reveal that the person is ready to move away from the conversation.
Foot direction	Foot direction indicates direction of interest	As mentioned, the knee and feet tend to point toward the focus of interest or away from people or things that are not interesting. In a group dynamic, if someone points her feet outward at a 45-degree angle, it means she is open to others joining her. When someone's feet are pointing toward each other, it suggests she is not open to others joining her.
Shoe play	Flirting, boredom, "My feet hurt!"	In certain situations, dangling our shoes from our feet or slipping our feet in and out of our shoes has a sexual overtone. Alternatively, it can convey boredom or simply indicate that our feet hurt.

Source: Adapted/paraphrased with permission from Businessballs.com (n.d.).

Personal Space

What is considered an "acceptable" amount of personal space between people depends on many variables, such as the culturally specific social norms, the situation at hand, personal preferences, and the nature of the relationship between those involved. Violations in personal space can cause friction, even if these violations are due simply to ignorance or a lack of spatial awareness. Hall (1966) states that there are five distinct space zones, as described in Table 2.8.

Table 2.8 The Five Space Zones

ZONE	DISTANCE	INDICATION	RATIONALE
Close intimate	0–6 inches	Lovers, married people	This often occurs when one is face to face with someone and likely to kiss.
Intimate	6–18 inches	Close relationships	This is appropriate for people in intimate relationships and close friendships. People who are not in such relationships often feel this degree of proximity is very invasive and even threatening. For both parties to feel comfortable, permission is often needed.
Personal	18 inches to 4 feet	Family, friends of significance	We can give a simple handshake in this zone, but then we need to take a step back.
Social	4–12 feet	Social or business casual	We can give a handshake in this zone if we reach in a little toward each other (and we don't have to step back).
Public	More than 12 feet	Private or ignoring	We do this when we are trying to avoid interaction with others who are nearby.

Source: Hall (1966)

Sometimes, people may "invade" your personal space to the point of making you extremely uncomfortable. When this unwelcome invasion is sexual in nature, this is known as sexual harassment. Sexual harassment is prohibited in the workplace, and anyone who feels they are a victim of sexual harassment may take legal action. Note, however, that many victims of sexual harassment may be fearful of retribution and may therefore choose to engage in this type of unwelcome interaction rather than cut it short—let alone take legal action—due to fear of retaliation, job loss, or even physical harm (Leskinen et al., 2011). Script 2.2 shows you how to address someone who may be making unwelcome advances.

Your Road Map: Improving Body Language Messaging and Interpretation

Improving your ability to interpret body language can help you identify what *isn't* being said. This is especially helpful when a dichotomy exists between someone's words and actions, as well as for ensuring your own messaging is consistent. Either way, a little knowledge about the subconscious can be extremely powerful! Here are a few tips and tricks to help you better understand what others may not be saying and to ensure you don't send mixed messages yourself:

- **Don't jump to conclusions.** Consider all verbal and nonverbal body language gestures before you make absolute inferences.
- **Motivate yourself.** Becoming better at reading and engaging in body language takes a great deal of time, effort, and dedication. You must be highly motivated and want to learn.
- **Practice.** Practice how you want to appear to others in both simulated (watch yourself in a mirror) and real-world environments (take mental notes in real-time conversations).
- **Know the "naughty bits" rule.** Consider how much of the pelvis area you are showing others or someone is showing you. Showing or not showing this region of the body indicates the level of confidence one has in the person or situation (Driver & van Aalst, 2010). For example, covering this area with one's hands (such as when standing with a hand-over-top-of-hand stance) may indicate that one is uncomfortable or apprehensive about something or someone.
- **Use the belly-button rule.** Driver & van Aalst (2010) explain that the position of one person's belly button in relation to another is a great indicator of their interest level. For example, if a person is talking to you but has his or her belly button turned toward someone or something else, they may not be as interested in your conversation as their words indicate. This helps you determine whether a person is truly engaged in your conversation.
- **Pay attention to inconsistencies.** Nonverbal communication should reinforce spoken communication. Try to identify when you are saying one thing but your body language is saying something else—for example, telling someone "yes" with words while shaking your head "no." This may indicate that you don't know how to say no.

SCRIPT 2.2

What to say when…

YOU ARE BEING SEXUALLY HARRASSED.

T
Time and place to talk

Choose an appropriate time and place for the conversation. Find a private setting where you can have an open and focused discussion without distractions.

> I need to talk to you about a serious matter, immediately and in private. Do you have a moment?

E
Explain and explore perspectives

Clearly and objectively explain the specific instances or observations where you have felt that you are not being treated fairly. Use concrete examples to support your concerns, ensuring that your feedback is specific and constructive.

> There are times I feel very uncomfortable around you, specifically when you touch my arms or constantly rub my shoulders when you're talking to me.

L
Listen to their perspective

Give the other person an opportunity to share their perspective and provide any explanation for their behavior. Practice active listening and seek to understand their side of the story.

Example A: Apologetic

> Wow, I didn't realize this would make you so uncomfortable. I am sorry.

> I accept your apology; however, there is no excuse for your behavior. I expect you will keep your hands to yourself from this point forward.

Example B: Underestimating

> Are you kidding me? You are taking this way out of context! Don't flatter yourself.

> I thought you might respond this way, so I have an outline prepared to take to HR.

L
Leverage shared values and lead the conversation forward

Remind the person of the shared goals or values within the context where you feel you are being treated unfairly. Emphasize the importance of fairness, equality, and collaboration to achieve mutual success.

Example A: Apologetic

> *I will be sure not to touch you again. I didn't realize this was an issue.*

> *Thank you. Please know, if you touch me inappropriately again, I will be handing HR a log of your prior behavior, including this conversation.*

Example B: Underestimating

> *Oh please. You have no evidence. It will be a 'he said, she said' issue.*

> *I'm going to let HR handle this. (Exit immediately.)*

> When I agree with what someone else is saying, I mirror their body position, tone of voice, and pace of speech. I believe this makes people feel understood and respected.

- **Be a copycat.** When we *mirror*, or copy, another's body language during a conversation, we establish rapport. Mirrored body language generates an unconscious feeling of affirmation, thereby encouraging feelings of trust and connecting people on another level (Businessballs, n.d.; Driver & van Aalst, 2010). When people display body language similar to our own, we unconsciously feel, "This person is very similar to me and agrees with me. I like this person because we are similar." The opposite effect applies when body language gestures are *not* mirrored. People feel less alike, making the engagement less comfortable. Each person senses conflict arising because unconscious signals are mismatched. Mismatched signals can translate into unconscious feelings of disconnect, discomfort, or even rejection. The unconscious mind may perceive, "This person is not like me. I feel defensive and cautious."

- **Know where to stand when you speak.** Be cognizant of your proximity to others when speaking to them, as well as the positioning of your eyes, hands, legs, mouth, and pelvis (Businessballs, n.d.; Driver & van Aalst, 2010).

- **Look people in the eye when you talk.** Maintain eye contact both when speaking and while listening.

- **Control your body position.** Try not to look uptight when nervous. At the same time, don't look like you're so relaxed that you're disinterested or completely shut down and unapproachable.

- **Read other people's body language.** You'll know the effect you're having on others if you examine their posture, fidgeting, or frowns. If you don't like or trust what someone is saying, home in on their micro-gestures, such as their feet placement, eye direction, and facial expressions. Micro-gestures include small gestures such as eyebrow lifts, mouth twitches, or even contracted pupils. They are unconscious gestures; they can't be controlled. This makes them extremely useful in reading body language.

- **Control your facial expressions.** Some people have better poker faces than others. Try not to roll your eyes upward or otherwise show that you're bored, angry, inappropriately amused, or even sad.

- **Trust your instincts.** Don't ignore your gut feelings. If you get the sense that someone isn't being honest or something isn't adding up, you may be picking up on a mismatch between verbal and nonverbal cues. Try to focus on the other person's motive for giving mismatched signals. Are they hiding something?

- **Defy deception.** Some people have the ability to artificially control their body language to give the impression they want to create at the time. For example, a firm handshake and direct eye contact are signals that can easily be faked (Businessballs, n.d.; Driver & van Aalst, 2010).

> Not all gestures match up with their "meaning." When interpreting body language, it helps to look for clusters of signals rather than relying on only one.

Pulling It All Together With the CAR Framework

Now that you have a solid understanding of what certain gestures may reveal and how you can use this information for improved conversations, let's use the CAR framework to organize what you've learned:

- **Consideration:** Assess several different body language gestures throughout the whole conversation and consider them as an aggregate rather than as one body part at a time.
- **Action or call to action:** List all the body language gestures you noted (either in yourself or in someone else) and compare them with the possible inferences described in the tables presented earlier in this chapter.
- **Return on investment:** Did the body language match up with the situation and with what was being said? If yes, your return on investment (ROI) was high. If no, use the Question-Wait-Question (QWQ) formula to ask more questions in a follow-up conversation. This formula promotes active listening because waiting (silence) encourages a person to speak or share more information. For example, when there is a pause during a conversation, we normally interpret this as our cue to speak. QWQ helps us avoid this tendency to make room for others to share more. Silence in conversations can be very awkward, so pausing can be an extremely effective way to motivate others to talk.

Time to Reflect

Imagine a conversation in the breakroom in which a male nurse is sitting across from a female nurse. His left arm is positioned across his body, with his left hand holding the elbow of his right arm, his right hand covering his neck, and his feet turned slightly away from the female nurse toward the window. The woman's feet are directly facing the man, and she appears to be offering him information. Without having any prior knowledge, based on body language alone, who do you think has control of this conversation? If you answered the female nurse, you are correct. Who do you think feels uncomfortable or threatened? If you answered the man, you are correct.

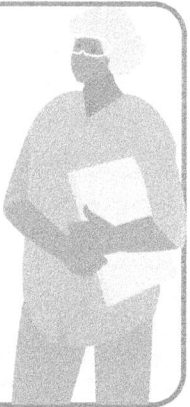

Body Language in Action

Whether I am presenting at a speaking engagement, caring for a patient, or coaching my staff, I remain aware of my body language. In many situations, certain circumstances warrant certain gestures. For example, if I have a large audience that I am about to speak to, I sometimes need to boost my confidence a tad. So, prior to walking on stage, I hold my body in the high-power pose—leaning back slightly to open my chest, placing my hands on my head with my elbows out—while taking a few slow breaths. This posture stimulates higher levels of testosterone—a hormone associated with power and dominance—in my body, while suppressing cortisol, a stress hormone. This reduces any stress or butterflies I may be experiencing prior to presenting.

When I want to motivate my patients, staff, or audience to participate in conversation, I listen! That means avoiding multitasking—for example, checking my watch, email, texts, or missed calls. I focus on them by directing my belly button and feet toward them and making eye contact. I am respectful of the distance I stand from them, and I lean toward them when possible. I nod occasionally, and I use head-tilt gestures to convey that I'm confused (eyes squinting) or I'm interested (eyes open and eyebrows raised). I hold my arms a little wider than my stance, and I never cross them in front of my chest unless I want to issue a nonverbal response to what I'm hearing.

To encourage collaboration in my conversations, I make sure there are no physical barriers between me and the other person—for example, a desk, a water cooler, or even a podium. When possible, I sit next to people at a safe distance. I don't cover my pelvis with my hands. If I am giving a presentation with slides, I hold the slide advancer to my side rather than across my body in a defensive or protective way. If I do have to hold something else, such as a chart or books, I make sure I hold it at waist level. (I feel that the closer people hold objects to their chest, the more insecure they appear.) I move my hands a lot when I speak—in an open manner, with forearms facing up, or steepling.

When I want to place emphasis on something I said, I pause and place my hands on my hips, in a Superman pose. Alternatively, as I walk around the room, I might lightly fold my hands in front of me, just above my belly but below my chest, parallel to my waist. I then bounce my folded hands up and down in the same rhythm as my speaking rhythm to emphasize important points. It's amazing the amount of emphasis you can place on your conversations by moving your hands! When addressing questions from a group, I make sure my feet are in a triangular position so that others feel welcomed into the conversation, as appropriate.

When having a conversation with someone new, I offer a genuine smile and a firm handshake with my palm facing to the side and a slight squeeze at the end as I repeat the person's name. Repeating their name is for my benefit, not theirs. I have a terrible memory, and repeating their name helps me remember it. (My poor memory is also why I rely so much on acronyms, as you'll see throughout this book!)

When my students carry a conversation too far, and I want to get their attention, I don't yell over them. Instead, I begin to speak while keeping my voice low. If I speak in an authoritative manner in the same monotone that I use when saying "um-hum" with my lips closed, I sound stern but not threatening. I get a better response with this approach than I do when I yell, "OK everyone, settle down!"

By focusing on both your verbal and nonverbal language when communicating with others, you can better direct the conversation to get the results you want. You have only a small window of opportunity to leave a good impression, so you must learn how to control your nonverbal gestures.

> Another trick I use to help with my memory is to make sure my arms and legs are unfolded when I'm listening. Pease and Pease (2008) found that when a group of volunteers sat with their arms and legs unfolded during a lecture, they remembered 38% more than a group that attended the same lecture and sat with folded arms and legs.

The Drive Home

Let's drive home the key points in this chapter:

- Body language can have different meanings to different people and in different settings.
- Just because someone looks to the left or to the right doesn't mean he is being creative or recalling facts, respectively. To make such an assessment, you must also consider all subtle and not-so-subtle hand, eye, and body gestures.
- Collecting and analyzing all body language cues provides a much more accurate depiction of what's *not* being said than focusing on one body gesture only.
- Interpreting body language is about being constantly mindful of the signals people give.
- Body language is not just about interpreting signals made by other people. It is also about gaining better self-awareness and self-control. Body language helps us understand thoughts and feelings in others *and* in ourselves.
- Being a copycat—also called mirroring—is not simply mimicking someone. Mirroring involves positioning your body to match another person's to help the person feel more comfortable around you.

References

Bolton, R., & Bolton, D. G. (2009). *People styles at work…and beyond: Making bad relationships good and good relationships better.* AMACOM.

Businessballs. (n.d). *Body language.* https://www.businessballs.com/self-awareness/body-language-70/

Driver, J., & van Aalst, M. (2010). *You say more than you think: A 7-day plan for using the new body language to get what you want.* Crown Publishers.

Goodreads. (n.d.). *Aristotle quotes.* https://www.goodreads.com/quotes/20103-the-whole-is-greater-thanthe-sum-of-its-parts

Hall, E. T. (1966). *The hidden dimension.* Anchor Books.

Leskinen, E. A., Cortina, L. M., & Kabat, D. B. (2011). Gender harassment: Broadening our understanding of sex-based harassment at work. *Law and Human Behavior, 35*(1), 25–39. https://doi.org/10.1007/s10979-010-9241-5

Mehrabian, A. (1972). *Nonverbal communication.* Transaction Publishers.

Mehrabian, A. (1980). *Silent messages: Implicit communication of emotions and attitudes.* Wadsworth Publishing Co.

Merrill, D. W., & Reid, R. H. (1981). *Personal styles and effective performance.* CRC Press.

Pease, B., & Pease, A. (2008). *The definitive book on body language: The hidden meaning behind people's gestures and expressions.* Bantam.

Tracom Group. (1991). *The social style profile–technical report: Development, reliability, and validity.* The Tracom Corporation.

3

The Emotionally Intelligent and Emotionally Competent Nurse

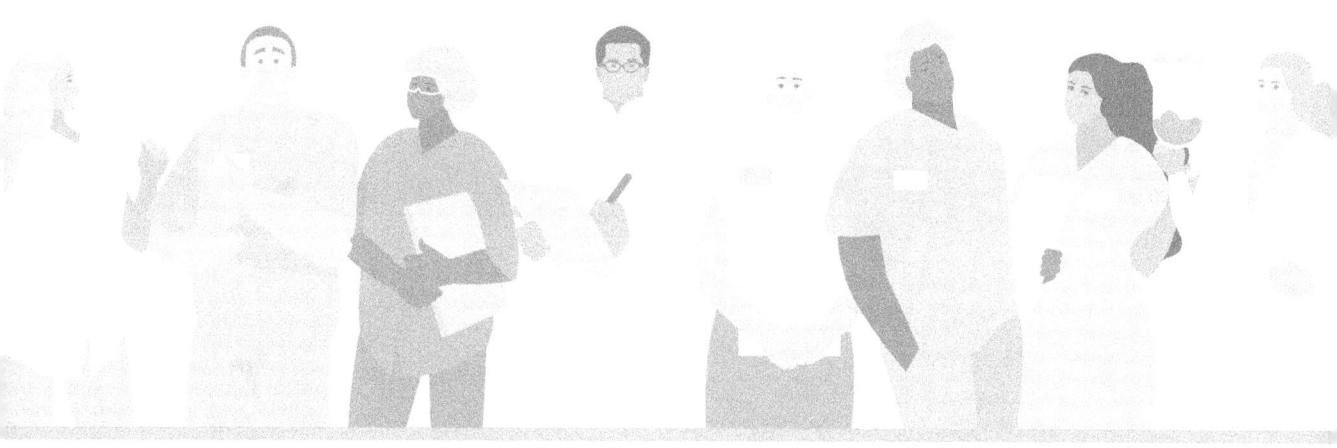

"Anyone can become angry. That is easy. But to be angry with the right person, to the right degree, at the right time, for the right purpose, and in the right way—that is not easy."

–Aristotle

Your emotions have a physical basis in the brain—which means that understanding how the brain processes emotions can help you understand them.

Figure 3.1 shows the parts of the brain that process emotions. This process works as follows (Goleman, 1998):

1. One of our five senses—sight, smell, taste, touch, or hearing—receives an external stimulus and sends a corresponding signal to the thalamus. The thalamus acts like an air traffic controller to keep the signal moving.

2. Typically, the signal is sent to the cortex, which deciphers, analyzes, and categorizes the signal and sends it to the neocortex.

3. The neocortex, which is the "thinking" brain that helps us solve problems, strategize, and analyze information, sends the signal to the amygdala.

4. The stimulation of the amygdala—the "emotional" brain—provokes an emotional response.

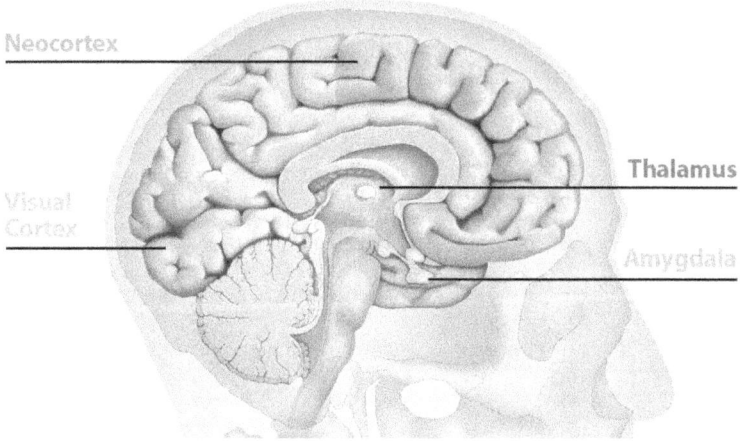

Figure 3.1 A simplified illustration of how the brain processes emotions.

The amygdala is the oldest, most primitive part of our brain. It organizes behavioral, autonomic, and hormonal responses to a variety of stimuli, including emotions that produce disgust, fear, or anger. It also plays a role in processing odors and pheromones, which are associated with sexual and maternal behaviors (Goleman, 1998).

The primary purpose of the amygdala is to keep us safe. It helps us avoid threats, protect ourselves from harm, and prepare ourselves for future dangers. The amygdala can respond to fear in as little as 0.07 seconds—which is why it is such an important part of our survival mechanism.

When our amygdala perceives a threat, it releases a stress hormone called *cortisol* into our prefrontal cortex (PFC). This prevents the PFC from operating at full capacity to manage complex processes like reason, logic, problem-solving, planning, and memory. Because we are so preoccupied by the threat, we can't think logically or rationally. Basically, the PFC shuts down—which is why this process is often called an *amygdala hijack*.

At the same time, the amygdala triggers a physiological response to the perceived threat, often called the *fight-or-flight response*. This response, also known as the *stress response*, occurs when we are in the presence of something we perceive as harmful—either mentally or physically. This response spurs us to either fight back against the perceived danger or flee it.

When you experience the fight-or-flight response, your body undergoes a number of changes:

- Your heart rate may increase.
- Your vision may narrow (aka "tunnel vision").
- Your muscles may become tense.
- You may begin to sweat.
- Your hearing may become more sensitive.

All these are adaptive bodily responses that help us stay safe. Because these responses are important to our survival, they occur quickly and without thought. They are automatic.

Imagine you are in the middle of a very stressful shift. Your unit is short-staffed, you've had issues with the pharmacy, and it seems like half of the equipment you need is missing. On top of that, you've worked 10 hours of your 12-hour shift without a break. In a word, you are exhausted. As you're trying to catch up on documentation and juggle other competing priorities, the call light for one of your patients—someone who just had leg surgery—goes off. When you walk into the patient's room, you immediately see that the portion of the patient's blanket that is covering his legs appears bright red. Before you can rationally assess the situation, your heart starts pumping hard and your body starts shaking. "Oh no!" you think, starting to panic. "The patient is bleeding out!" By the time you calm yourself down and grasp what's happened—someone spilled a large cup of red juice on the patient—you realize that the patient, who was resting comfortably before you entered the room, is now just as panicked as you are because of your response. This is a perfect example of an amygdala hijack.

The good news is that you can learn to manage and regulate your emotions to avoid responding to situations like these in an irrational manner. This will help you stay poised and under control (Goleman, 1998). This practice is one aspect of something called *emotional intelligence* (EI). Daniel Goleman identifies five key aspects of EI:

- **Self-awareness:** This describes your ability to understand, recognize, and identify your moods, drives, and emotions. Good leaders are also aware of how their demeanor affects others.
- **Self-regulation:** Not everything we desire is beneficial. Hence, self-regulation is an important aspect of EI. Examples of self-regulation include behaviors such as thinking before acting or speaking.
- **Internal motivation:** Success in and of itself can be an emotionally empty goal. Internal motivation indicates something deeper. A desire to do good, a willingness to go the extra mile, and remaining optimistic in the face of failure are good examples of internal motivation.
- **Empathy:** This refers to the ability to understand other people's emotional states and connect with them where they are. (This is different from sympathy, which implies concern or pity.)
- **Social skills:** These are what we use to build and enhance relationships. They are essential for leadership, for team-building, and for life.

The study of EI pulls from numerous segments of emotional, behavioral, and communications theories, including neuro-linguistic programming. EI in nursing contributes to better patient outcomes and emphasizes the need for continuous training and education to enhance EI skills (Bru-Luna et al., 2021; Khademi et al., 2021). Having a high EI helps us become more productive and efficient—and helps others do the same. Finally, a high EI can help us decrease workplace bullying and violence (Dellasega & Volpe, 2013). For example, an emotionally intelligent person is less apt to lash out at someone—even if that someone is yelling at them. This is because people with high EI are aware of their feelings, and this awareness checks the temptation to yell back.

In the Driver's Seat: Understanding Your Emotions and Your Intelligence

Lazarus (1991) describes emotions as brief events or "episodes" that we direct toward someone or something in response to how we feel about a person, a situation, an experience, or an outcome. We experience joy, fear, anger, and other emotional episodes in response to tasks, customers, coworkers, patients, or even something like a new electronic medical record.

Emotions can change our physiological state—for example, elevating or lowering our blood pressure or heart rate or causing us to perspire. They can also affect our behavior. Behavioral effects of emotions might include changes to our facial expression, tone of voice, and eye movement. These reactions are involuntary and often occur unconsciously. (See Chapter 2 for more information.)

Working With People Means Working With Emotions

We all come to work dealing with emotions that stem from situations in our personal lives. These emotions can include anger, sadness, and joy, to name a few. Some nurses can set these emotions aside and prevent them from interfering with new emotions they experience during their workday. Other nurses lack this ability.

There are limitations to each approach. For example, if a nurse shows up to work angry because her husband forgot to take out the trash, and now their garage will stink horrifically for the party she's planned for the upcoming weekend, she may displace this anger by yelling at a colleague about something she would normally have been more rational about. On the other hand, if a nurse leaves her anger behind, she may appear rigid or stoic when a colleague comes to her about some other issue.

Increasing EI in the healthcare setting means acknowledging that emotions will always surface and that you not only need to be aware of them but also need to do something smart with them. People vary immensely in the skill with which they react to and use their emotions as well as the emotions of others.

This skill is particularly important for those in leadership positions. For example, a unit nurse leader who has genius-level IV skills or critical-thinking skills but lacks EI may have trouble effectively managing staff. Research supports the notion that high EI correlates strongly with transformational leadership styles. Indeed, leaders with high EI give extra effort, perform better, feel less personally depleted, and experience greater overall satisfaction (Taylor et al., 2015; Tyczkowski et al., 2015).

Negative emotions often permeate healthcare organizations. These negative emotions can be contagious and can metastasize throughout the organization more quickly than you can take someone's pulse. It's important to learn how to cope with such feelings. Identifying what situations typically cause you to experience negative emotions enables you to implement a strategy to disrupt the cycle.

The REAL WORLD

Saikia et al. (2023) published a study that suggests EI training for nurses can be an effective way to improve the healthy workplace environment in healthcare organizations. EI training can include training in self-awareness, self-regulation, empathy, social skills, and motivation. Specific training techniques may also include role-playing exercises, group discussions, and individual coaching or mentoring.

The Need for Emotional Competency

EI is the ability to identify emotions. Having EI isn't enough, however. In addition to having EI, you must also have *emotional competence* (EC). EC refers to an ability to express emotions in real time and to connect consistently and effectively with others (Goleman, 1998). In other words, EC is the application of EI.

EI and EC are very powerful because they help you stay in control of your emotions. Although your subconscious is automated to provide immediate responses, your conscious mind can redirect these responses to be more positive. People with high EI and EC manage their emotions well, communicate effectively, lead change, solve problems, and use humor to build rapport when faced with adversity. They also embody empathy, exude optimism, and can educate and influence others. Finally, they have a unique ability to maintain their composure in chaotic situations—a quality that often separates high performers from low performers.

Recall the social styles discussed in Chapter 1: driving, amiable, analytical, and expressive. People who have EI are aware of these different social styles. People who have both EI and EC not only know about these styles; they apply certain techniques to cultivate better relationships with people who exhibit each style. These techniques are listed in Table 3.1.

Table 3.1 Using the Social Style Model to Foster Relationships

SOCIAL STYLE	HOW TO CONNECT BETTER WITH THIS GROUP
Driving	Allow them control in decision-making. Focus on results and efficiency. Remain objective.
Amiable	Be sensitive. Be sensitive to them. Ask them open-ended questions. Otherwise, they will try to answer you based on how you want them to answer.

SOCIAL STYLE	HOW TO CONNECT BETTER WITH THIS GROUP
Analytical	Provide factual and detailed information. Don't rush them. Support their reasoning.
Expressive	Express enthusiasm. Be accepting of the relationship they are trying to build with you. Give compliments and praise.

Sources: Merrill & Reid (1981); Tracom Group (n.d.)

The Impact of EI and EC on the Healthcare Environment

Using EI and EC in a healthcare environment is vital. One obvious reason for this is that it provides an awareness of the importance of introspection. Another perhaps less obvious reason is that there is a link between EI (and EC) and employee retention and good fiscal stewardship (Godse & Thingujam, 2010). According to the Health Resources and Services Administration (2022), there is a projected shortage of 78,610 full-time equivalent (FTE) RNs in 2025 and a shortage of 63,720 FTE RNs in 2030.

If it costs up to $100,000 to recruit, orient, and backfill a nursing position with overtime or agency use (depending on the specialty), then a hospital staffed with 200 nurses can expect to spend millions per year on new hires (Blake, 2006). An EC and stress-reduction program can cut turnover substantially (Cherniss & Goleman, 2001; Jha & Bhattacharya, 2021). Indeed, EC is reported to be a better predictor of workplace success and should be counted more heavily than intellectual ability (Goleman, 2005).

Research has revealed the following EI and EC success stories:

- According to the Hay Group (n.d.), 44 Fortune 500 companies discovered that salespeople who scored high in EI had twice as much revenue as those with mediocre EI scores.
- Rozell and colleagues (2002) found a correlation between EI and work performance in a sample of people who sold medical devices. In this study, EI was a reliable predictor of high work performance.
- Within 18 months of implementing EI assessments, a large metropolitan hospital decreased critical care nursing attrition from 65% to 15% (Petrides & Sevdalis, 2010).
- The Johnson & Johnson Consumer & Personal Care Group surveyed 358 of its managers globally to determine whether certain leadership skills or competencies differentiated high-performing managers from average ones. Results of this study demonstrated that managers with high EI performed better than others (Cavallo & Brienza, 2001).

The Relationship Between Emotional Intelligence and Nurse-Nurse Collaboration

A study examined the correlation between EI and collaboration among nurses and investigated how nurses' EI abilities impacted their ability to effectively work together in a collaborative environment. The research highlighted that nurses with higher levels of EI demonstrate enhanced communication skills, empathy, and conflict resolution abilities, which contribute to improved collaboration among their peers. By fostering EI skills, such as self-awareness and social skills, healthcare organizations can promote a positive work culture, enhance teamwork, and ultimately improve patient outcomes. The study emphasized the importance of recognizing and developing EI in nursing practice to enhance nurse-nurse collaboration. (Al-Hamdan et al., 2021)

Measuring EI

Several tests are available to measure EI, each focusing on different aspects. These include the following:

- **Emotional and Social Competency Inventory (ESCI):** This test, administered by the Hay Group, is the latest version of the Emotional Competency Inventory (ECI) by Richard Boyatzis and Daniel Goleman (Six Seconds, 2011). It uses Goleman's model to measure a spectrum of critical competencies shown to affect workplace performance. The ECSI is a multi-rater, so the test-taker receives feedback from several people.

- **Mayer-Salovey-Caruso Emotional Intelligence Test (MSCEIT):** This test measures one's ability to identify, use, understand, know, and solve emotional problems by asking a series of objective questions. It measures the intelligence behind the emotions of perceiving, using, understanding, and managing feelings. This is considered an "ability test"—in other words, it evaluates responses according to correctness rather than self-assessments (Six Seconds, 2011).

- **Six Seconds Emotional Intelligence Test (SEI):** This test measures eight basic EI skills, including emotional literacy, navigating emotions, intrinsic motivation, and empathy (Six Seconds, 2011, para. 5).

- **Emotional Quotient Inventory 2.0 (EQ-i 2.0):** This test is a newer tool based on the EQ-i by Reuven Bar-On. It measures self-perception, self-expression, decision-making, and stress management.

EI Versus the Myers-Briggs Type Indicator

Emotions, thoughts, and behaviors determine a person's unique personality. Personality describes how one operates—for example, whether they prefer to be around people. It does not, however, measure EI or identify thinking patterns the way EI does (Goleman, 2005).

The Myers-Briggs Type Indicator (MBTI) is a test that measures certain aspects of a person's personality. To achieve this, the MBTI uses four psychological scales (Myers et al., 1998):

- **Extroversion–Introversion:** This describes an individual's energy flow. Extroverts are charged up by being actively involved in events. They enjoy action, and they make things happen. They also enjoy being around people, and they energize others. Finally, extroverts understand a problem more efficiently when they can talk about it out loud and when others share their thoughts and perceptions. In contrast, introverts prefer self-examination and self-discovery. These individuals tend to conceal their feelings. Introverts prefer to work alone, and they learn better by watching others rather than participating (Myers et al., 1998).

- **Sensing–Intuition:** This describes how an individual learns. Sensors use their five senses to understand things. They learn best when they can see the pragmatic aspects of the matter at hand, and they relish real-life examples and hands-on applications. Intuitive people rely on their gut instincts—an unconscious reasoning that propels them to act without telling them why or how. They learn based on their feelings. Intuitive people tend to use their imagination to understand and learn (Myers et al., 1998).

- **Thinking–Feeling:** This describes how an individual makes decisions and choices. Thinkers use logic, objective principles, and impersonal facts. They ask the question "Why?" and analyze the pros and cons of each possible answer. Thinking people also tend to be consistent and logical in their decision-making. In contrast, feelers prefer harmony and do their best to help others. They make their best decisions by weighing what other people care about and always consider others' points of view (Myers et al., 1998).

- **Judging–Perceiving:** This describes how an individual deals with the world. Judgers prefer an orderly way of life and like to have things settled and organized. They like control, structure, rules, and organization. Perceivers prefer a flexible and spontaneous way of life. They like to understand and adapt to situations rather than organize them. Perceiving people are flexible, open to new experiences, and like to explore (Myers et al., 1998).

MBTI personality tests typically distinguish only these four categories of temperament. They do not measure behavior. Consider a scenario in which a nurse is interviewing for a sales position for a medical device company. The owner of the medical sales company knows he wants a nurse with an extroverted personality to fill the sales position, but he can't distinguish from a temperament test which nurse will be perceived as *persistent* (a positive quality that describes someone with energy, drive, and a thick skin, which is helpful for developing new business) and which will be perceived as *insistent* (who may be perceived as pushy).

Here's another example: Suppose you need to hire a nurse for a role that requires one to have the characteristics of an extrovert, sensor, thinker, and judger (ESTJ). According to the MBTI, such a person will be outgoing, pragmatic, consistent, and logical. However, the MBTI will not indicate how the person will behave under stress.

Simply put, we can't predict behaviors based on personalities. We all know people who are fun, energetic, and outgoing. These qualities do not necessarily equate with success in the workplace, however. Even people who are energetic and fun can make errors in judgment regarding their behavior. Consider a nurse leader who is typically fun and energetic but breaks down and acts aggressively when someone or something goes awry. It's crazy how quickly some nurse leaders transition from the good to the bad to the ugly—without giving the rest of us any time to take cover! This can turn an organization's culture of safety into a culture of fear. (This example also helps explain why people with similar personality styles can't necessarily perform the same job successfully.)

Just as one's MBTI personality type does not offer insight into one's behavior, it does not indicate one's level of EI or EC (Thompson, 2006). Personality and EI are different. A person's personality is a structured set of distinctive features or characteristics that make that person unique within their thoughts, inspiration, and actions in different conditions. In contrast, EI refers to a person's ability to manage their emotions and the emotions of others to reach a desired outcome.

> ## Time to Reflect
>
> As a staff nurse, manager, or nurse executive, you might have asked yourself some of the following questions:
>
> - Why do certain nurses seem to get into more accidents than others?
> - Why do some nurses ignore organizational policies and procedures?
> - Why do some nurses use illegal drugs during work?
> - Why do some nurses cause confrontations and problems?
> - Why do some nurses achieve high patient experience scores, while other clinically competent nurses struggle to build any type of rapport with their patients?
>
> In many cases, the answers to these questions relate to the nurse's EI and EC rather than their personality type.

Your Road Map: Improving Your EI and EC

Unlike our intelligence quotient (IQ), which peaks around age 17 and remains constant throughout adulthood, we can continually develop our EI. In fact, according to Sze and colleagues (2012), our EI can rise steadily during adulthood. Research also shows that the presence of EI (or lack thereof) can predict a person's work performance and level of career success (Goleman, 1998).

The EQ-i model posits that the best way to increase EI is to build on existing strengths rather than to focus on rectifying deficits (Joseph & Newman, 2010). Let's first look at ways to improve EI and EC. We'll then look at some ways to control common emotions.

Improving EI and EC

Improving EI and EC involves improving the following:

- **Self-awareness:** To improve your self-awareness, try the following:
    - **Journal your feelings.** This simple act can improve not just your self-awareness but your mood, too.
    - **Slow down.** When you experience a strong emotion, try to slow down. Examine what exactly triggered the emotion. Although you can't control the situation, you can control your reaction to it.
- **Self-regulation:** Here are a few ways to improve self-regulation:
    - **Know your values.** What values are most relevant to you? On what values are you unwilling to compromise? Examine your own personal code of ethics. Understanding what is most important to you will help you make good choices.
    - **Hold yourself accountable and own your problems.** Don't blame other people for your problems. Make a commitment to admit mistakes and accept consequences. In addition to helping you take responsibility for yourself, this practice will earn you the respect of others.
    - **Practice being calm.** The next time you find yourself in a challenging situation, be aware of how you act. Practice deep-breathing exercises and think through your emotions.
- **Motivation:** To improve motivation, try the following:
    - **Reexamine why you're a nurse.** When faced with adversity, it's easy to forget what you really love about nursing. When this happens, reflect on why you went into the nursing profession in the first place. This may help you view your situation in a more positive light.

- **Know where you stand.** Look in the mirror and determine how motivated you are to lead change. Think about what motivates you and how you can motivate others.
- **Be encouraging.** Motivated nurses remain positive, no matter what challenges they face. The next time you are confronted with an issue, problem, or failure, try to find something positive about it—even if it's something trivial or small.
- **Social awareness:** To improve your social awareness, consider the following tips:
  - **Put yourself in someone else's shoes.** Consider situations from other people's perspective. This can shed a completely different light on things and allow for conflict resolution.
  - **Pay attention to body language.** A person's body language can reveal how they *really* feel about a situation. As a nurse, being able to read body language can be a real asset because you can glean how someone feels without their disclosing it. (For more information on body language, see Chapter 2.)
  - **Respond to other's feelings.** Suppose you ask a nurse colleague on an earlier shift to stay on to cover you because you're running late for work. Although she agrees, you can hear the disappointment in her voice. Respond by addressing her feelings. Tell her you appreciate that she is willing to stay for you and that you're just as upset about being late. Promise to pay it forward when she needs you—and keep your word.
- **Relationship management:** To improve relationship management, try the following:
  - **Learn to resolve conflict.** Nurses must know how to resolve conflicts between colleagues, patients, and doctors. Demonstrating conflict-resolution skills can halt gossip, backstabbing, and other toxic behaviors. This skill is vital if you want to succeed in any area of nursing. See Script 3.1 for a way to handle gossiping in the workplace.
  - **Recognize the accomplishments of others.** Recognizing and sharing accomplishments with your patients, colleagues, and leaders, as appropriate, can go a long way toward building relationships. Remember: Commend in public and coach in private.
  - **Improve your communication skills.** The next time you're in a conversation, pay attention to how much you're listening compared to how much you're speaking. One way to do this is to apply the Question-Wait-Question (QWQ) formula, discussed in the nearby sidebar.

The Question-Wait-Question (QWQ) Formula

This helpful formula, introduced by Driver (2010), ensures there is two-way communication by encouraging you to use active listening and encouraging the other person to share more information. Powerful people acknowledge that sharing too much personal knowledge can make them look weak, so they encourage others to speak more than them (Driver, 2010).

Maria Shriver (2012) spoke of the "power of the pause" at the University of Southern California's Annenberg School commencement ceremony. She explained that we need to pause in conversations to learn more from others. Instead of stepping on other people's words, try breathing and listening more (Driver & van Aalst, 2010).

In addition to urging her audience to take a pause during conversations to allow others to speak, Shriver suggested they:

> Have the courage to press the pause button…Whenever you are in doubt, pause. Take a moment. Look at all of your options. Check your intention. Have a conversation with your heart. And then always take the high road. (Shriver, 2012)

The QWQ format and Shriver's "power of the pause" represent a superlative approach to self-management. Anytime you stop to assess what you're feeling, you raise your self-awareness, enhance your relationships, and increase your ability to make a positive difference.

Controlling Common Emotions

Some emotions, such as frustration, worry, anger, dislike, and disappointment, are hard to overcome, but you can do it if you consistently work through them. Let's review strategies to overcome these complex emotions.

SCRIPT 3.1

What to say when…

YOU NEED TO ASK A COLLEAGUE TO STOP GOSSIPING.

T

Time and place to talk

Choose an appropriate time and place for the conversation. Find a private setting where you can have a focused discussion without distractions.

Example: Coworker

> Colin, do you have a minute? I need to speak with you in private. Someone is going around the unit telling everyone that I'm dating our new surgeon, Dr. Pete.

E

Explain and explore perspectives

Clearly and objectively explain the specific instances or observations where you have noticed your colleague engaging in gossip. Use concrete examples to support your concerns, ensuring that your feedback is specific and constructive.

Example A: Playing Dumb

> I have no idea what you're talking about.

> I wish whoever is saying this would stop. Can you help me in stopping this?

Example B: Confrontational

> It's no big deal.

> This may be true, but it's no one's business. We don't have the right to share each other's private information.

Example C: Defensive

> Do you know who is telling everyone?

> It doesn't matter who; I just need the gossip to stop.

L
Listen to their perspective

Actively listen and try to not make assumptions. Focus on looking at the big picture to gain more insight.

Example A: Playing Dumb

> Wow, that's a shame. Sorry to hear this, but there is nothing I can do.

If you hear someone saying this, I really need you to tell them it's none of their business and to stop spreading gossip.

Example B: Confrontational

> There are bigger issues at hand. Your love life isn't so important. Don't worry about gossip.

We need to respect each other's privacy.

Example C: Defensive

> Sorry, I don't have anything to do with it.

Well, if you know who is spreading the gossip, it would really mean a lot to me if you would tell them to stop.

L
Leverage shared values and lead the conversation forward

Give your colleague an opportunity to share their perspective and provide any explanation for their behavior. Practice active listening and seek to understand their side of the story.

Remind your colleague of the shared goals or values within the workplace. Emphasize the importance of fostering a positive and supportive work environment, where trust and professionalism are prioritized.

Example: Playing Dumb/Confrontational/Defensive

I'm sure this wasn't done maliciously, but I'd appreciate your help in stopping the gossip. If it continues, I will need to take further action and report that I'm being harassed.

Dealing With Frustration

Frustration usually occurs when one feels stuck or trapped. For example, suppose you just arrived at work, and a patient or family member rudely confronts you about a problem that occurred before you arrived. It can be very frustrating to try to fix a problem that you had nothing to do with! Still, keeping your frustration level at a minimum is key to optimal outcomes. Here's how:

- **Stop**. Stop and ask yourself why you feel frustrated. Be clear and specific about the source of your angst. If needed, write down your answer. This allows you to assess the situation. When you're finished, think of one positive thing about your situation. For instance, if a doctor placed you on hold for a long time, then a positive aspect of the situation might be that you had extra time to prepare your question(s) for the call or even that you got to stand still for a few moments. This positive way of thinking can improve your mood greatly.

- **Reflect.** Recall the last time you were frustrated by someone or something. Ask yourself: Did your frustration solve your problem? Probably not. Then move forward, not backward. There is no point in doing otherwise.

Handling Worry

Nurses have lots of causes for worry. They often care for very sick patients and are frequently asked to do more with less. This worry can easily spiral out of control if you allow it—affecting not only your mental health but also your productivity. Try these tips to overcome worry:

- **Remove yourself from the situation.** For example, if nurses start to gossip about impending layoffs, avoid the conversation so you won't worry with them.

- **Breathe.** Take five deep breaths, breathing in through your nose and out through your mouth. Each breath should take approximately five seconds. This technique will help slow your breathing and your heart rate and lower your anxiety.

- **Concentrate on actions.** If you fear being laid off, don't sit and worry. Instead, show how valuable you are by brainstorming and helping to implement ideas.

- **Start a "worry log."** Use a notebook to document situations that worry you, and schedule time to deal with them later. This enables you to put the worries to the side and focus on other important issues. When it comes time to deal with the worries, try to identify patterns and take action to break them.

One cause of worry is overwork. Script 3.2 provides a sample conversation you might have when asking your supervisor for help with your workload.

Managing Anger

For various reasons, many nurses experience anger in the workplace. Anger is a destructive emotion that becomes even more toxic when it is mismanaged. Nurses often take their anger out on each other, which causes even more harm (Dellasega & Volpe, 2013). If you have trouble managing your temper at work, then learning to control it is one of the best things you can do—especially if you want to keep your job and your sanity. Try these suggestions from Dellasega and Volpe (2013) to control your anger:

- **Watch for early signs of anger.** Learn to recognize when your anger is building as soon as it begins.
- **Stay in control.** Even if you can't change what's making you angry, you can choose how you react to something or someone that angers you—and your best choice is to stay in control. You can't help becoming angry, but you can deflect your anger and remain in control!
- **Take a break.** Shut your eyes for a few minutes and take some deep breaths. This will interrupt your angry thoughts and place you on a more positive path.
- **Look in a mirror.** Think about how and what you look like when you're angry. Is this how you want others to see you? Would you want to interact with someone who looks this way? Probably not.

Of course, you're not the only person who gets angry at work. See Script 3.3 for how to deal with someone else who is angry.

SCRIPT 3.2

What to say when…

YOU NEED TO ASK YOUR SUPERVISOR FOR HELP WITH YOUR WORKLOAD.

T
Time and place to talk

Find an appropriate time and place to have a conversation with your supervisor. Choose a moment when they are available and not too busy, and ensure you have their full attention.

Example: Nurse Manager

> *Beverly, I am realizing my eagerness to 'do more' has gotten the best of me. I would like to speak with you to discuss some solutions. When can we meet?*

E
Explain and explore perspectives

Clearly and objectively explain the challenges you are facing with your workload. Provide specific examples and details about the tasks or responsibilities that are overwhelming you.

Example A: Understanding

> *I appreciated your eagerness to help out. What are your thoughts?*

> *First, I would like your help in setting priorities on each project.*

Example B: Disappointed

> *What? I was really counting on you to help me out. I should have known you would drop the ball.*

> *I have accepted more than I can handle, and it is important to me that I sustain my typical high performance. There is just more work than hours in the day. I don't believe this is because of my inability. I believe it is the workload. You may not be aware that my current responsibilities include …*

L
Listen to their perspective

Allow your supervisor to share their perspective and insights. Be open to their suggestions or recommendations on how to address the workload issue. Practice active listening and seek to understand their point of view.

Example A: Open to Suggestions

> Where do we begin?

> I would like your help in setting priorities on each project. I would also like to incorporate some other staff members to take accountability on the projects. If everyone pitches in, we can obtain more creativity and have a better chance at meeting our deadline.

Example B: Disappointed

> So I guess this is just another mess for me to clean up?

> I can arrange a meeting on Monday to discuss the projects with the group and take the lead in delegating to staff.

L
Leverage shared values and lead the conversation forward

Emphasize that your goal is to perform your duties effectively and contribute to the overall success of the team or organization. Highlight the importance of maintaining quality work and meeting deadlines to support the team's objectives.

Example A: Receptive

> I'm glad you brought this to my attention.

> I would like to express my thankfulness for your support.

Example B: Unreceptive

> Are you sure you can at least handle that?

> I am working beyond full capacity, where safety and quality could be compromised. I would like to think you would appreciate that I recognize my own strengths and weaknesses. This has been a learning opportunity for me, and your support would be appreciated.

Dislike

Sadly, we have all worked with someone we didn't like. Whether it was their attitude, their work ethic, or even the amount of perfume they wore (see Script 3.4), it is often tough to work with certain types of people. Fortunately, with the right strategies, you can still have a productive working relationship with someone you dislike:

- **Be respectful.** Take the higher road and treat the person you dislike with basic respect and courtesy.
- **Be mindful.** Figure out why you don't like this person. Is it their behavior? Who they hang with in the breakroom? The tone of their voice? Then think about why you have these feelings. Although there is no simple solution to dealing with dislike, bringing mindfulness to the process can help.
- **Be empathetic.** Whatever the reason for your dislike of someone, remember: You're in control of how you react to them. Put yourself in their shoes. When you do, you'll realize they—like most people—probably aren't trying to be difficult, unkind, stubborn, or unreasonable; they're simply reacting to the situation through their own lens.

Disappointment

If you've just suffered a major disappointment, such as negative comments from your nurse manager during your annual work evaluation, it's easy to get down on yourself. This may prevent you from going above and beyond in the care of your patients. Here are some proactive steps you can take to cope with disappointment:

- **Know your core values.** Take a moment to consider what values are most important to you. Are you disappointed because you violated your own core values or because you feel you let someone or something else violate your core values?
- **Respond early.** If your gut tells you that you need some space away from someone or something, take it. Once you have space, reflect on things that make you happy. This reflection won't necessarily make you happy instantaneously, but it will help you think about more positive things than what is disappointing you at the moment.

In addition, consider having a conversation with your manager, as shown in Script 3.5.

Time to Reflect

Two nurses on different units each had an argument with their boss at work. On returning home, the first nurse, who lacked EI, started shouting at her kids because they were arguing with each other. She didn't realize that this outburst was really a displacement of her feelings about the argument she had with her boss. She demonstrated low EI.

When the second nurse returned home and found that her kids were arguing, she thought, "Why should I shout at the kids? They are not the ones to blame for my feelings. The main reason I am feeling badly is because of the argument at work, not my kids." The second nurse recognized her emotions, thought about them, and acted in an emotionally intelligent way.

Which of these nurses would make a better leader?

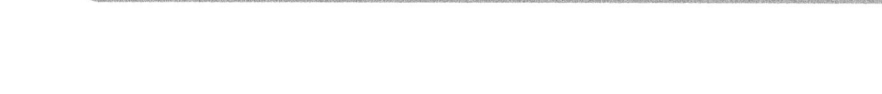

Improving Your Leadership Skills

According to Goleman (2004), leadership skills—unlike innate academic or technical aptitude—are learned in life. If you are a weak leader, you can, with the right effort, improve at virtually any point in your life. Getting better requires motivation, a clear idea of what you need to improve, and consistent practice.

For example, suppose you need to develop your listening skills—an important quality of any good leader. Maybe you have a habit of interrupting people mid-sentence or even completely hijacking conversations. The first step to improving your listening skills is to become aware of when you do this and stop yourself immediately. (Review the QWQ formula from earlier in this chapter.) Or maybe you have to deal with someone who constantly interrupts you. This can be incredibly annoying, but if you control your emotions, you will better be able to help the person eliminate this behavior. See Script 3.6 for an example of how you might address such a situation.

Another skill that good leaders possess is the ability to help others stay positive. Leaders who attain the best results get people to laugh three times more often than mediocre leaders do (Goleman et al., 2002). Because laughter signals relaxation and enjoyment, this suggests that people who laugh often are more likely to be focused and productive.

SCRIPT 3.3

What to say when…

YOU NEED TO DEAL WITH AN ANGRY PHYSICIAN.

T

Time and place to talk

Find an appropriate time and place to address the situation. Choose a moment when both you and the physician can have a private and uninterrupted conversation.

Example: Physician

> Dr. Chou, I am aware you are angry with surgical throughput. (Allow him to vent and then restate the issue in a simplified manner.) So, if I understand you correctly, you are frustrated because we have been running behind on our surgical cases all week.

E

Explain and explore perspectives

Clearly and calmly explain the specific incident or issue that has caused the physician's anger. Stick to the facts and avoid making personal judgments or accusations.

Example A: Rational

> Yes, I just want organization and timeliness in my OR.

> I appreciate your concern. I understand that delays in surgical cases cause a lot of issues. I want to find a remedy also.

Example B: Angry

> Yes, my OR times should not be so convoluted. You need to get your act together and fix this.

> I appreciate your concern. I understand that delays in surgical cases cause a lot of issues. But your anger toward me is not the answer to this problem. We need to work together, not against each other.

L
Listen to their perspective

Allow the physician to express their thoughts and emotions. Practice active listening and avoid interrupting. Let them fully explain their viewpoint and concerns.

Example A: Apologetic

> Look, I know you're trying, but it's all very frustrating that something so easy is so difficult around here.

> I will contact these departments and see if there is a simplified approach; if not, I will arrange meetings. I know you're busy. I'd really appreciate your support on this.

Example B: Angry

> I'm here to operate, not to play cruise director.

> There are multiple touch points where the cases are backing up. We need to work with housekeeping, admissions, and transport to improve the throughput. I will contact these departments and see if there is a simplified approach; if not, I will arrange meetings. Your presence is key to moving this forward. Can I count on you as part of this team approach?

L
Leverage shared values and lead the conversation forward

Emphasize the common goal of providing the best possible care to patients. Remind the physician that effective collaboration and respectful communication are essential in achieving positive outcomes.

Example A: Supportive

> Start making the calls. Let me know what I need to do.

> I will start making the calls after our last case today. I am looking forward to working with you on this.

Example B: Unsupportive

> Why do I have to do everything? What do they pay you to do around here, anyway?

> I will start making the calls after our last case today. If you can support me on this, we will have a more productive outcome. I will not tolerate your outbursts and will contact the leadership team on how to proceed in this. I hope you will reconsider working with me.

SCRIPT 3.4

What to say when…

YOU NEED TO TAKE THE "FUMES" OUT OF A COLLEAGUE WEARING TOO MUCH PERFUME/COLOGNE.

T
Time and place to talk

Find an appropriate time and place to have a private conversation with your colleague. Choose a moment when they are not engaged in any urgent tasks and when you can have their undivided attention.

Example: Colleague

Hi Juanita, I'd like to ask you something in private. Do you have a moment? (When in private, continue.) If I wore too much perfume, would you tell me?

E
Explain and explore perspectives

Clearly and tactfully explain the concern you have regarding the amount of perfume your colleague is wearing. Focus on the impact it has on you or others in the workplace, rather than making personal judgments.

Example A: Doesn't Take the Hint

Yes, I'd tell you, why do you ask?

Well, I appreciate that, and that's why I wanted to bring this to your attention. I find your perfume strong and thought you might want to know.

Example B: Takes the Hint

Yes. Are you saying I am wearing too much?

Yes, and I thought you might want to know, just as I would want someone to tell me.

L
Listen to their perspective

Give your colleague an opportunity to share their perspective and any reasons behind their choice of wearing a strong perfume. Practice active listening and seek to understand their viewpoint without judgment.

Example A: Offended

> You should really mind your own business.

> I don't mean to cross the line. I just thought if I mentioned this, you might wear less. I'm sure you are not aware how strong the scent is, but I thought you'd rather hear this from me than from others. You're not alone. We all have times when we aren't aware that we put too much on.

Example B: Embarrassed

> I spilled it, and it ran all over my clothes. That's why it's so strong.

> I understand. It happens. please be sure to let me know if I'm ever wearing too much, too, OK?

L
Leverage shared values and lead the conversation forward

Remind your colleague of the shared goals or values within the workplace, such as promoting a comfortable and respectful environment for all employees. Emphasize the importance of considering the impact of one's actions on others.

Example A: Offended

> I know how much and what I put on my body. Maybe you should pay more attention to the outfits you wear than my scent!

> I am respectful to you and ask that you are respectful to me by not wearing such a strong perfume. It is giving me headaches. If you don't, I will have to take this issue to our manager.

Example B: Embarrassed

> I probably won't wear any tomorrow!

> I'm glad we're able to have open discussions like this. Thank you for understanding.

SCRIPT 3.5

What to say when…

YOU WANT TO OPTIMIZE YOUR ANNUAL EVALUATION.

T
Time and place to talk

Begin by discussing your key accomplishments and contributions as a nurse. Highlight specific instances where you provided exceptional patient care, improved outcomes, or went above and beyond your duties. Provide concrete examples and outcomes to support your claims.

Example: Nurse Manager

> *I enjoy what I do, and I am looking forward to reviewing my performance with you.*

E
Explain and explore perspectives

Discuss your core nursing competencies and strengths that have positively impacted your performance. Highlight any professional development or certifications you have pursued during the year. Emphasize how these strengths have improved patient outcomes and contributed to a positive work environment.

Example A: Negative

> *I have concerns about your work performance, specifically your tardiness. If you continue to be late, you will lose your job!*

> *Agree: I understand, and I'm ready to work on an action plan.*

> *Disagree: I don't understand how you came to this. Could you elaborate?*

Example B: Positive

> *I have been really impressed by your work ethic this past year.*

> *Thank you for the recognition of my hard work.*

L
Listen to their perspective

Share your short-term and long-term goals as a nurse. Discuss your desire to further develop your skills, take on leadership responsibilities, or contribute to quality improvement initiatives. Demonstrate your commitment to ongoing professional growth and your dedication to providing excellent patient care.

Example A: Understanding

Agree: I will make sure I clock in on time, which is only up to seven minutes before the time of my shift; otherwise, I am considered late. And if I clock out seven minutes after my shift is over, I understand that is unapproved overtime, and I am subject to disciplinary action.

Disagree: Can you show me how many times I was actually late?

Example B: Goal Setting

I want to continue to work hard, and I would appreciate your support in allowing me to take some management courses next year to be considered for promotion.

L
Leverage shared values and lead the conversation forward

Based on your accomplishments, strengths, and goals, propose any specific actions or opportunities you would like to explore to further excel in your role. This could include additional training, participation in research projects, or involvement in committees or initiatives.

Example A: Negative

I expect more from you. I expect you to be on time.

Agree: I understand if I continue to be late or go into overtime, you will need to start formal disciplinary actions.

Disagree: I will expect then for you to contact me when I am not in compliance since I don't see this reflected on the time clock.

Example B: Positive

I will be happy to sign you up for some professional development courses.

Thank you for your support. I'm looking forward to another great year.

Nurse leaders rarely fail in the workplace because they lack clinical skills. Rather, many nurse leaders fail because of emotional shortcomings that lead to a loss of trust in their relationships with others. These shortcomings might include autocratic tendencies, an inability to reduce conflict, a tendency to promote a culture of fear, and the assumption that everyone shares their perceptions. Regarding this last point, many people assume that what is good for them must be good for others. For example, because most people in leadership positions are driven to excel, they often assume that all employees are similarly wired. Leaders with strong EI and EC understand that these types of biases and perceptions are just that—and *not* objective reality.

Understanding the Oz Principle

Connors et al. (2010) introduced the Oz principle, which is based on the moral of the movie *The Wizard of Oz*. According to the Oz principle, organizations can be crippled when employees see themselves as victims and play the blame game instead of practicing accountability. This principle, or philosophy, propels staff to overcome adversity to achieve the results they desire by being accountable for their actions.

Like Dorothy's search for the Wizard of Oz for guidance, staff also look for a "wizard" to rescue them from problems and conflicts at work. The connection between *The Wizard of Oz* and these workplace issues is that, in both cases, there *is* no wizard. There's just the ugly truth—which, in a healthcare setting, is often a lack of individual and/or organizational accountability. When problems in this setting are not addressed, a toxic cycle of blame, overlook, and ignorance often festers, and no improvements are made.

People with high EI and EC own accountability and manage issues using the following approach (Connors et al., 2010):

1. **See it:** The first step is to acknowledge there is a problem.

2. **Own it:** This means to take responsibility for the problem.

3. **Solve it:** Next, the person takes steps to find solutions to the problem.

4. **Do it:** In this last step, the person drives the implementation of the solution(s) identified, while also being cognizant of behaviors and emotions in themselves and others.

Some key aspects of the Oz principle include the following:

- **Beware of victimization.** Just as Glinda, the good witch from *The Wizard of Oz*, explained to Dorothy that she always had the power to find her way back home, you always have the power to stay in control of your emotions—especially when faced with adversity such as gossip. Do not fall victim to following the yellow brick road in hopes a wizard will fix all your problems! Remember: Even when you feel powerless, you do have choices. You gain nothing from feeling as if you're a victim of circumstance. As long as you recognize that you are choosing to do something—whether staying in a job you don't enjoy or doing nothing at all—you can reclaim your power (Connors et al., 2010).

- **Take control.** If you come into the workplace with a poor attitude, or you always see "them" (that is, executive leadership or any other group with decision-making power) as wrong and you as right, you are the one at fault. Attitude is a matter of perspective—and perspective is significant. As discussed in the book *The Oz Principle*, hold yourself accountable in situations by asking yourself, "What else can I do to achieve the results I desire or overcome the circumstance that plagues me?" (Connors et al., 2010). In other words, it's not always "them"—and even if it is, the power to change your negative thoughts into positive ones is within your control.

- **Being right isn't what is most important.** Focus less on being right all the time and more on being perceived as someone who helps, promotes solution-oriented problem-solving, and gets things done. You don't have to be right every time to be perceived as effective and appreciated—but you do have to be helpful!

The Drive Home

Let's drive home the key points in this chapter:

- Goleman (1998) identified the five key domains of EI as self-awareness, self-regulation and management, motivation, social awareness, and relationship management.

- Signals from our five senses that involve emotion are sent to the amygdala, which is the brain's emotional command center. The amygdala organizes behavioral, autonomic, and hormonal responses to a variety of situations, including emotions that produce disgust, fear, and anger.

- It is very important to be aware of what you are feeling. For example, you must be able to identify when you are on the verge of losing control of your emotions.

- Feelings have an impact on just about everyone we interact with. Nurses need to be able to read emotional cues from patients, colleagues, and staff.

- Controlling your emotions requires you to be empathetic to others. You need to be able to relate to what others are feeling. This will help you better understand them.

SCRIPT 3.6

What to say when…

YOU NEED TO CONFRONT A HABITUAL INTERRUPTER.

T

Time and place to talk

Choose an appropriate time and place to address the issue. Find a moment when both you and the person you are speaking to can have a private and uninterrupted conversation.

Example: Coworker

> Paige, I have a problem I'd like your help with. Do you have a moment to talk in private?

E

Explain and explore perspectives

Clearly and assertively explain that you would like to be heard without interruptions. Express the importance of having a respectful and uninterrupted conversation to ensure effective communication.

Example A: Receptive

> Sure, what's up?

> When I talk, I like to get to my point, but I find it difficult when I can't finish my sentences. Although I do appreciate your insight, it's when you chime in while I'm in mid-sentence that I easily lose track of where I was going with the conversation to begin with.

Example B: Defensive

> I'm really busy. I can't help you.

> This will only take a few minutes. I'd really appreciate your time. Look, when I talk, I like to get to my point, but I find it difficult when I can't finish my sentences. Although I do appreciate your insight, it's when you chime in while I'm mid-sentence that I easily lose track of where I was going with the conversation to begin with.

L
Listen to their perspective

Allow the person to share their thoughts and perspectives on the matter. Practice active listening and give them the chance to express any concerns or reasons behind their interruptions. Show that you value their input while also asserting your need to be heard.

Example A: Receptive

> I didn't realize I did that to you. I guess I do this a lot?

> I'm noticing a pattern more and more and thought I should bring this to your attention.

Example B: Defensive

> Are you seriously taking up my time to tell me this?

> When I am energetic about other people's conversations, I've noticed that I also chime in too early, and I'm trying to wait for pauses before I express my thoughts. I'd really appreciate it if you could help me do this, and I can offer you the same—if you're accepting.

L
Leverage shared values and lead the conversation forward

Emphasize the importance of open and respectful communication in achieving shared goals. Remind the person that interrupting can hinder effective collaboration and understanding.

Example A: Apologetic

> I am sorry. I don't even know I'm doing this until after I do it and only when there is a look of awkwardness on the person I interrupted!

> What if when I see that you are ready to chime in too early, I hold up my finger in a 'wait your turn' fashion, but discreetly, of course?

Example B: Denial

> I think you are just oversensitive.

> Paige, you interrupted me yesterday during the safety huddle. I was ready to explain how many patients left the ED before being seen, but before I could give the stats, you interjected with how full the ICU was. If you continue to interrupt me, I'm going to announce that you are interrupting me in our next conversation so that you'll become more aware of this.

References

Al-Hamdan, Z. M., Alyahia, M., Al-Maaitah, R., Alhamdan, M., Faouri, I., Al-Smadi, A. M., & Bawadi, H. (2021). The relationship between emotional intelligence and nurse–nurse collaboration. *Journal of Nursing Scholarship, 53*, 615–622. https://doi.org/10.1111/jnu.12687

Blake, R. (2006). *Employee retention: What employee turnover really costs your company.* https://www.studocu.com/en-us/document/university-of-arkansas-at-little-rock/team-development/employee-retention-what-it-really-costs-your-company/34612693

Bru-Luna L, M., Martí-Vilar M., Merino-Soto C., & Cervera-Santiago J. L. (2021). Emotional intelligence measures: A systematic review. *Healthcare, 9*(12). https://doi.org/10.3390/healthcare9121696.

Cavallo, K., & Brienza, D. (2001). *Emotional competence and leadership excellence at Johnson & Johnson: The Emotional Intelligence and Leadership Study.* http://www.eiconsortium.org/reports/jj_ei_study.html

Cherniss, C., & Goleman, D. (Eds.). (2001). *The emotionally intelligent workplace: How to select for, measure, and improve emotional intelligence in individuals, groups, and organizations.* Jossey-Bass.

Connors, R., Smith, T., & Hickman, C. (2010). *The Oz principle: Getting results through individual and organizational accountability.* Portfolio.

Dellasega, C., & Volpe, R. L. (2013). *Toxic nursing: Managing bullying, bad attitudes, and total turmoil.* Sigma Theta Tau International.

Driver, J. (2010). *You say more than you think: A 7-day plan for using the new body language to get what you want.* Crown Archetype.

Godse, A. S., & Thingujam, N. S. (2010). Perceived emotional intelligence and conflict resolution styles among information technology professionals: Testing the mediating role of personality. *Singapore Management Review, 32*(1), 69–83.

Goleman, D. (1998). *Working with emotional intelligence.* Bloomsbury Publishing.

Goleman, D. (2004, January). What makes a leader? *Harvard Business Review.* https://hbr.org/2004/01/what-makes-a-leader

Goleman, D. (2005). *Emotional intelligence: Why it can matter more than IQ.* Random House.

Goleman, D., Boyzatzis, R., & McKee, A. (2002). *Primal leadership: Realizing the power of emotional intelligence.* Harvard Business Press.

Hay Group. (n.d.). *Leadership transformation.* https://www.haygroup.com/uk/services/index.aspx?id=2490

Health Resources and Services Administration. (2022). *Nursing workforce projections, 2020–2035.* https://bhw.hrsa.gov/sites/default/files/bureau-health-workforce/Nursing-Workforce-Projections-Factsheet.pdf

Jha, P., & Bhattacharya, S. (2021). The impact of emotional intelligence and servant leadership on employee job satisfaction. *International Journal of Innovation Science, 13*(2), 205–217. https://doi.org/10.1108/IJIS-09-2020-0169

Joseph, D. L., & Newman, D. A. (2010). Emotional intelligence: An integrative meta-analysis and cascading model. *Journal of Applied Psychology, 95*(1), 54–78. https://doi.org/10.1037/a0017286

Khademi, E., Abdi, M., Saeidi, M., Piri, S., & Mohammadian, R. (2021, July 20). Emotional intelligence and quality of nursing care: A need for continuous professional development. *Iran Journal of Nursing & Midwifery Research, 26*(4), 361–367. https://www.ncbi.nlm.nih.gov/pmc/articles/PMC8344623/

Lazarus, R. S. (1991). *Emotion & adaptation.* Oxford University Press.

Merrill, D. W., & Reid, R. H. (1981). *Personal styles and effective performance.* CRC Press.

Myers, I. B., McCaulley, M., Quenk, N., & Hammer, A. L. (1998). *MBTI handbook: A guide to the development and use of the Myers-Briggs Type Indicator* (3rd ed.). Consulting Psychologists Press.

Petrides, K. V., & Sevdalis, N. (2010). Emotional intelligence and nursing: Comment on Bulmer-Smith, Profetto-McGrath, & Cummings (2009). *International Journal of Nursing Studies, 47*(4), 526–528.

Rozell, E. J., Pettijohn, C. E., & Parker, R. S. (2002). An empirical evaluation of emotional intelligence: The impact on management development. *Journal of Management Development, 21*(4), 272–289.

Saikia, M., George, L. S., Unnikrishnan, B., Nayak, B. S., & Ravishankar, N. (2023). Thirty years of emotional intelligence: A scoping review of emotional intelligence training programme among nurses. *International Nursing Review.* Advance online publication. https://doi.org/10.1111/inm.13235

Shriver, M. (2012). *USC Annenberg School of Communication commencement speech* [Video]. https://www.youtube.com/watch?v=A5xLcLIlXqU

Six Seconds. (2011). *Six Seconds Emotional Intelligence Assessment (SEI)*. http://www.6seconds.org/tools/sei/

Sze, J. A., Goodkind, M. S., Gyurak, A., & Levenson, R. W. (2012). Aging and emotion recognition: Not just a losing matter. *Psychology and Aging, 27*(4), 940–950. https://doi.org/10.1037/a0029367

Taylor, B., Roberts, S., Smyth, T., & Tulloch, M. (2015). Nurse managers' strategies for feeling less drained by their work: An action research and reflection project for developing emotional intelligence. *Journal of Nursing Management, 23*(7), 879-887. https://doi.org/10.1111/jonm.12229

Thompson, H. L. (2006). Exploring the interface of the type and emotional intelligence landscapes. *Bulletin of Psychological Type, (29)*3, 14-19. https://hpsys.com/PDFs/Type_%20and_EI_Landscapes2.pdf

Tracom Group. (n.d.). *The social style model*. https://www.tracomcorp.com/social-style-training/model/

Tyczkowski, B., Vandenhouten, C., Reilly, J., Bansal, G., Kubsch, S. M., & Jakkola, R. (2015). Emotional intelligence (EI) and nursing leadership styles among nurse managers. *Nursing Administration Quarterly, 39*(2), 172-180. https://doi.org/10.1097/NAQ.0000000000000094

4
Mindful Conversations

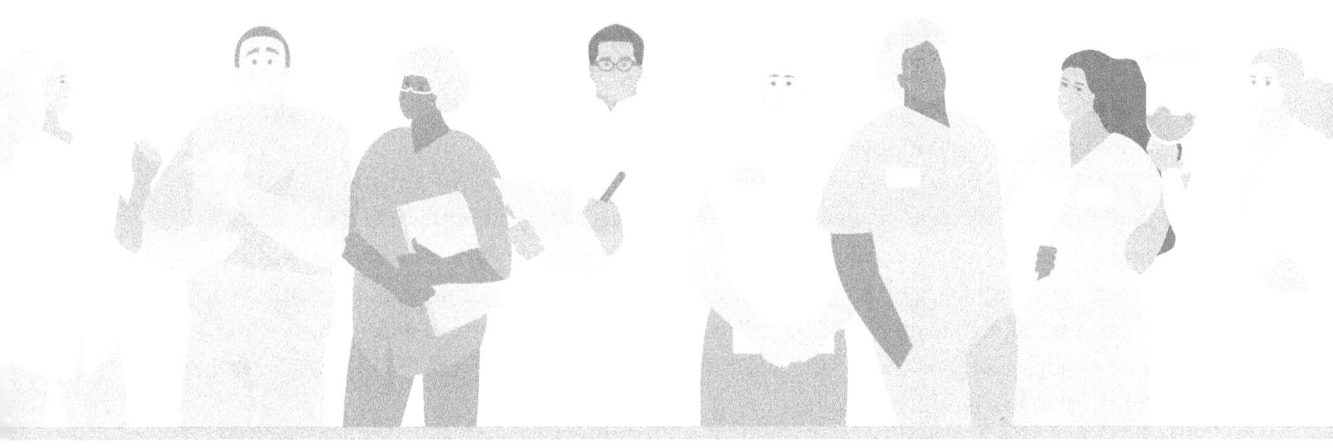

"Do not dwell in the past, do not dream of the future, concentrate the mind on the present moment."
–Buddha

One day, my son came home from school and told me he had won a contest. I was very proud of him, and I wanted to listen—but I also needed to dig through several emails, and I continued to do so as he spoke. It wasn't until he stopped mid-sentence that I realized that my inattention had hurt his feelings. "Continue the story!" I said, mustering my enthusiasm. "No," he said sadly, "I get it. Your email is more important than I am." Talk about a wake-up call! That very moment I vowed to be more present—more mindful—when communicating with others.

Mindfulness is about being present in whatever is happening in the present moment (Kabat-Zinn, 1994). Dr. Jon Kabat-Zinn at the University of Massachusetts defines *mindfulness* as "paying attention in a particular way: on purpose, in the present moment, and without judgment" (Mindful, 2017, para. 2).

Mindful communication involves conversing with kindness, attention, and compassion. It means maintaining an intentional focus or awareness on the current state as well as a growth mindset. When we communicate mindfully, we are cognizant of our emotions, thoughts, and environment. This helps us translate our thoughts into meaningful and respectful words. It also demonstrates sensitivity to others. Mindful communication enables us to remain open to multiple points of view and to understand things in new ways.

With mindful communication, people feel heard, understood, and empowered (Kabat-Zinn, 1994). This is due in large part to the active listening required by mindful communication. Listening—*really* listening—is one of the greatest gifts we can give someone. Listening with intention shows that we care. It also improves our social awareness—our sense of people's moods, behaviors, and motives.

Mindful communication involves more than listening and speaking clearly. It also involves using nonverbal communication. Our body language often reveals more than we realize. Through mindfulness, we become more aware of what we communicate nonverbally. When we are mindful, we are more thoughtful about how our body gestures make other people feel. Being mindful about our body language helps us become more aware of how we affect other people, as well as how they affect us.

Mindful communication enables us to improve our conversations, influence others, make good decisions, and manage expectations. Moreover, it doesn't take any more time than "regular" communication, and it doesn't require the person with whom you're talking to be versed in it. Simply having this skill set ourselves enables us to lead conversations in a positive direction (Kabat-Zinn, 1994; Taren et al., 2015).

A Taste of Mindfulness

I recently attended a mindfulness course for healthcare providers. This course served as an introduction to the theory, practice, and application of mindfulness. It taught me several simple practices that I now use with clients and patients.

The course included both didactic content and experiential learning. Whereas the didactic content emphasized current research about the benefits of mindfulness-based interventions, the experiential modules offered an introduction to key mindfulness practices for reducing stress and enhancing therapeutic presence (Jefferson Health, 2017).

One piece of the experiential learning involved mindful eating. More specifically, it involved eating a raisin. Sounds simple enough, right? Just eat a raisin. As it turned out, however, this exercise was not as simple as it sounded. Yes, eating a raisin is quite simple in theory. But *mindfully* eating a raisin is much more complex.

The instructor began the exercise by asking us to set an intention: specifically, to bring an open mind to the experience of eating a raisin. She then asked us to put aside all distractions—including turning off our phones—and to focus on clear awareness of each aspect of the experience.

The instructor gave each of us a cup containing three raisins and asked us to focus on just one. "Look at the raisin as if you've never seen anything like it before," she advised. She told us to notice the folds in the raisin, where the surface of the raisin reflected light or appeared darker, and any asymmetries or unique features. Just as I thought to myself, "Why am I doing this?" the instructor calmly told us to acknowledge any thoughts we were having about the exercise by letting them be and to then bring our awareness back to the raisin.

Next, the instructor asked us to pluck a raisin from the cup and hold it in the palm of our hand or between our finger and thumb. She told us to explore its texture and urged us to close our eyes to enhance our sense of touch. We then were instructed to hold the raisin beneath our nose, and with each inhalation, to drink in any smell, aroma, or fragrance that arose. As I did this, I noticed some sensations in my mouth, and I began to salivate. I couldn't believe I was salivating over a dried-up, sad-looking raisin. I don't even *like* raisins! Finally, our instructor asked us to bring the raisin to one ear, squeeze it, roll it around, and see if we could hear any sound coming from it. (Note that I did not hear a sound coming from the raisin—although I did hear plenty of self-talk asking what I was doing listening to a raisin!)

At last, our instructor told us to slowly bring the raisin to our lips. As we did so, she asked us to notice how our hand and arm knew precisely how and where to position the raisin. Then she told us to gently place the raisin in our mouth, without chewing it. I could taste the raisin and feel its various textures with my tongue. She told us to chew the raisin and to detect when we felt ready to swallow it. Finally, she instructed us to swallow the raisin and to focus on how it felt as the raisin moved down our throat and into our esophagus on its journey to our stomach. When it was all over, I considered how my body as a whole felt after completing this exercise.

This experience helped me put into perspective what it really meant to be mindful. It helped me see that focusing is hard—especially with so many other thoughts pinballing around my brain—and that this is both natural and OK. I simply had to permit myself to focus on what I was experiencing while eating the raisin in that moment.

In the Driver's Seat: Be Mindful, Not Mind Full

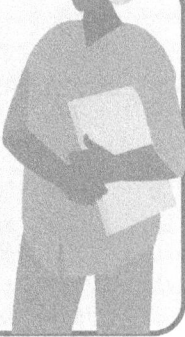

Being mindful can improve communication, enrich collaborations, boost our emotional intelligence, promote innovation, and facilitate decision-making. But these days, it seems as if our minds are just too *full* to be mindful. High-speed technology, coupled with our ultra-short attention spans and our constant need to multitask, make it hard enough to complete a thought, let alone a task! As a result, we often engage in conversations that are misunderstood, misused, or mismanaged.

> **Time to Reflect**
>
> Have you ever practiced mindful eating? How did it affect your experience of the meal? How could you apply what you've learned from mindful eating to other aspects of your life?

Feeling constantly under stress from our daily routines—such as getting the kids off to school, commuting to work, fielding countless emails and text messages, struggling to meet tight deadlines, and so on—means we are constantly in fight-or-flight mode. The fight-or-flight instinct is good if we are in real peril—say, face to face with a saber-toothed tiger. But it's bad when we exist in this mode all the time. This is because the fight-or-flight instinct makes it impossible to remain calm and rational. Our fight-or-flight reflex often causes us to freak out—to become overwhelmed by emotion—which often places us in challenging or awkward situations.

Because we convey our innermost feelings, beliefs, and thoughts to the outside world through communication, it's important to understand the role our emotions play in the words we choose. Emotionally challenging situations can cause our thoughts to become so twisted up that we not only grow confused about what we want to say but also lose track of our words, pitch, tone, and inflection. As a result, we may appear hostile, scattered, or confused to the people with whom we are trying to communicate—which in turn leaves us feeling misunderstood, misrepresented, and even downright frustrated. Practicing mindfulness gives us a much better chance of being heard and understood, as well as allowing us to better understand others (Basso et al., 2019).

The Neuroscience Behind Fight-or-Flight

The fight-or-flight instinct is triggered by the *amygdala*—the structure in the brain responsible for our emotional responses. When we sense danger, the amygdala becomes hyper-engaged. This causes us to lose access to our frontal lobe, which controls important functions such as problem-solving, memory, language, emotional regulation, judgment, decision-making, and attention.

The good news is that we can tame our primal responses to stress by employing Mindfulness-Based Stress Reduction (MBSR) or even daily mindfulness meditation. MBSR is a group program developed by Jon Kabat-Zinn during the 1970s to help patients struggling with life's difficulties (Kabat-Zinn, 1994). Although it was initially formed to help patients in the hospital, it now has widespread applicability and has been used by people from all walks of life.

Mindfulness strengthens our relaxation response and decreases stress hormones, such as cortisol. Mindfulness also increases the concentration of our gray matter. The more gray matter we have, the better we are at evaluating rewards, consequences, and overall thought processes. Finally, it increases both the activity and the size of the prefrontal cortex, which is part of the frontal lobe (Goleman, 2005).

Research in neuroscience shows that our minds are as malleable as our bodies (Taren, 2015). Practicing mindfulness or participating in MBSR can help you train your mind in the same way exercise can train your body.

Feeding the Right Wolf

There's an old Native American story—variously attributed to the Cherokee and the Lenape tribes—about a grandfather speaking to his grandson about inner conflicts. "In each human heart," says the grandfather, "there are two wolves battling one another. One is fearful and angry. The other is understanding and kind."

"Which one will win?" the young boy asks his grandfather.

"That's simple," the grandfather says. "Whichever one we choose to feed."

When we experience negative emotions such as hurt, anger, and fear, it is often easier to feed the fearful, angry wolf. Indeed, these robust and intolerable negative feelings often follow pathways that become deeply ingrained in our nervous system—instantly rushing through us anytime our experiences trigger them. Negativity and stress hijack our emotions (Goleman, 2005) and attention. The result is poor behaviors—for example, using unkind words, slamming doors, sending scathing emails, or speaking ill of someone behind their back—and diminished outcomes.

Becoming more mindful enables us to disrupt this negative cycle. Through mindfulness, we can feed the wolf that is understanding and kind—and enjoy significantly improved outcomes.

Accepting Ourselves

You'll find as you practice mindfulness that your mind may still wander. When that happens to you, try not to judge yourself. It's only natural that your mind will do this. After all, we can listen much faster than others can talk! Our thoughts naturally turn to what's on our to-do list or how we can fix the other person's problem. Mindfulness practice teaches us to accept when we realize our mind has begun to wander and to give ourselves permission to return to a state of mindfulness.

Sometimes, when your mind wanders, it may meander into some pretty negative terrain—for example, thinking about someone who has hurt you and plotting your revenge. This is natural. It doesn't mean you're a horrible person. When these thoughts come into your mind, simply accept them and think them through. For example, if you feel yourself becoming angry with someone, simply notice that sensation, and remember that you need to cool down before you speak up and say something you might regret later.

Suppose you're upset with a coworker because she didn't stand up for you in a meeting. You've spent days—maybe even weeks—feeling angry. Without you necessarily being aware of it, your emotions may affect how you've been communicating with that person. Odds are she can sense your negative attitude toward her and may become defensive. The result is a vicious cycle of distressing feelings and resentment on both sides.

> It takes patience and practice to conduct an intelligent conversation without those maddening emotions hijacking your discussion! (Goleman, 2005)

Practicing mindfulness helps us become more cognizant of the fluctuations in our mood. Acknowledging our feelings—and approaching the situation from a place of honesty—helps us release resentment (Bru-Luna et al., 2021). For example, saying to yourself, "I feel angry and disrespected because my coworker didn't stand up for me during the meeting" will help you recognize your feelings and thereby clarify your mindset. This in turn helps you make more rational decisions and engage in more productive conversations.

Understanding Your Intention and Taming Your Tone

In addition to being mindful of our feelings, we must become mindful of our *intention*—that is, what we hope to accomplish—in any communication. Your intention will drive the direction of the conversation (or, in some cases, help you determine whether you should have the conversation at all).

Let's go back to the example of the coworker who didn't support you in your meeting. Is your intention in communicating with that person to make her feel bad? Or is it to try to resolve the issue? If your intention is to make her feel bad, you should wait until your emotions cool down to act. Odds are, when that happens, your intention will change to reaching a resolution.

Assuming your intention is one worth acting on—in this case, reaching a resolution—your next step is to focus your attention in a way that supports your intention. For example, if your intention is to have a level-headed conversation with someone to resolve a problem, then you should consider what words to use to meet your objective. This requires you to first crystallize in your mind exactly what you're thinking and feeling so you can successfully communicate this to others. Ask yourself, "How do I wish to express myself?" This will help you clarify what you value and how you would like to communicate it.

> It's important to stay open-minded even when we feel upset because there is always the possibility we misunderstood something. Misunderstandings happen, and we can better position ourselves for positive outcomes when we approach them with mindfulness, curiosity, and empathy.

Our words have a huge effect on how others perceive us. So, too, does our tone. Indeed, our tone can be even more powerful than our words. Like a chameleon, our tone can change depending on the environment. For example, we might start a conversation using a very diplomatic tone. However, if we sense that the other person is becoming defensive or exhibiting negative behaviors—in other words, the environment is changing—our tone can reflect this, often without our knowledge! Becoming aware of this changing environment the instant it shifts can help you maintain control of your tone to keep the conversation on point.

Time to Reflect

One aspect of tone is the pace of your speech. The next time you have a discussion with a family member or friend, try matching the pace of their speech. Then subtly change the pace of *your* speech—speaking either more or less slowly—to see if the other person follows you. Try this a few times to see what happens (but not in an obvious way).

Being Present

The goal of mindfulness is to be present in the moment—to simply notice with no thought or judgment, and without jumping into planning mode. Being present means:

- Acknowledging that something you said may need clarification
- Ensuring that the intention behind your words is understood
- Stating your intention instead of assuming others know what it is
- Using respectable words and an appropriate tone

> Mindful communication isn't about ignoring our emotions or acting stoic. It's about acknowledging and understanding how we feel, why we feel it, and how we convey our thoughts and feelings to others.

Time to Reflect

How mindful are you during conversations? Consider whether you fall into any of the following patterns when someone is speaking to you:

- You formulate your response even before the person has finished talking.
- Your mind wanders off to other things.
- You feel impatient.
- You complete their sentences.
- You interject your own related experience without validating what they are saying.

Chances are you have experienced at least one of these communication patterns. Remember, wandering is natural and simply tells us we have an opportunity to come back to the present. Being present allows us to better listen to what the person is saying, rather than assuming.

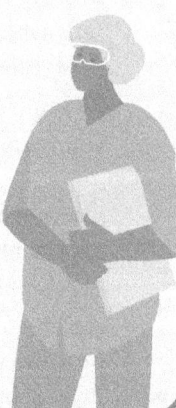

The REAL WORLD

At the Mindful Leader Summit in October 2022, there was great discussion on the benefits of practicing mindfulness in the workplace, the impact of mindful leadership, practical aspects of creating a culture of wellness across all industries, and how such a culture can lead to both corporate and personal success.

Mindfulness is becoming mainstream: Top companies are already prioritizing and implementing mindfulness training for employees. Many companies consider a mindfulness program an investment in learning and development. Some of the inspiring companies include Google, Toyota Motor Corporation, SXSW, Boeing, Lender Toolkit, SLB, Humana, and Nike.

Your Road Map: Communicating Mindfully

To communicate mindfully, you must be present. That is, you must remain in the moment by focusing on the situation at hand. This sets the foundation for productive dialogue. Remember, the greatest gift you can give others is to be present when they speak. The following strategies can help you be more present in conversations:

- **Adjust your mindset.** Before exchanging words, you must be in the right mindset. That is, you must enter the conversation with an open mind and be cognizant of the emotions you are experiencing. Approach the conversation with the intention to understand.
- **Eliminate distractions.** Where you place your attention will shape what you experience. Eliminate as many distractions as possible. Don't multitask.
- **Listen.** Ask yourself, "What matters most in this conversation?" This helps you get to the underlying values and needs in a situation and fosters understanding, collaboration, and problem-solving.
- **Be aware of body language.** Be aware of the other person's body language as well as your own. As discussed in Chapter 2, body language can often reveal more than just the words used.
- **Breathe.** Take a pause by being mindful of each inhalation and exhalation. This helps you relax and also helps oxygenate your prefrontal cortex—the rational part of your brain.
- **Show empathy.** Put yourself in someone else's shoes. This will help you understand things from their perspective and eliminate any judgment.
- **Show understanding.** When others share their thoughts and feelings, show them you understand by stating, "I understand," or, "I see what you mean." This gives them a sense of comfort that their words and feelings are relatable.
- **Paraphrase.** Paraphrasing what you heard enables you to clarify your understanding and convey to the person that you are listening.
- **Ask open-ended questions.** This helps solidify your knowledge and provides you with a deeper understanding of the conversation.

There are various courses and training that teach mindfulness. I highly recommend attending one to gain more insights into and appreciation for this practice. But you don't have to take a course to practice mindfulness. You can start today by taking just a few basic steps at the beginning or end of your day or whenever you need a boost:

1. Sit in a quiet area with both feet on the ground, hands resting freely on your lap or at your side.

2. Bring awareness to a specific area of your body—for example, your feet.

3. Notice your feet and how they feel pressed to the floor.

4. Stretch out your toes and then relax them. Notice the sensation. Notice the difference.

5. As your mind wanders, allow yourself to bring your attention back to the sensation of your feet.

When you feel comfortable with this exercise, you can add awareness to your ankles. Again, experiment with stretching and relaxing them. Then move slowly up your body, systematically bringing your attention to each area.

At first, practice mindfulness for two minutes at a time. Over time, increase the duration of each practice to 10 minutes. Research shows that practicing mindfulness for just 10 minutes per day for eight weeks has a long-lasting positive effect at the neurological level (Basso et al., 2019).

The REAL WORLD

A study of more than 100 General Mills directors and managers conducted by the Institute for Mindful Leadership (n.d.) found the following results on the effectiveness of mindful leadership after mindfulness training:

- 48% increase in ability to focus
- 40% increase in personal productivity
- 34% increase in ability to prioritize
- 31% increase in employee satisfaction
- 34% increase in ability to perform under pressure

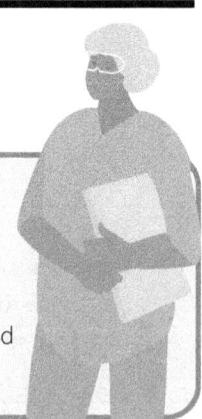

Time to Reflect

Think about something that happened during your day—anything at all. Notice whether, as you think about this event, your mind begins to wander. It most likely will. Then notice how many times your mind wanders during a five-minute period. How did you bring yourself back to what happened during your day?

The Drive Home

Let's drive home the key points in this chapter:

- Mindfulness helps us reach positive outcomes with our conversations.
- Mindfulness skills develop and enhance our emotional intelligence, decision-making, communication, innovation, and collaboration.
- Mindfulness and mindful communication help us ensure that others feel heard, understood, and empowered.
- The first step to a mindful conversation is to crystallize what we're thinking and feeling.
- Being present when we speak with others is the greatest gift we can give them.
- Practicing mindfulness can help us become more cognizant of the fluctuations in our mood, acknowledge our feelings, and approach the situation with honesty, which in turn helps us release resentment.
- Our intention drives the direction of our conversation.
- Our primal responses to stress can be tamed and more thoughtful responses achieved when we practice mindfulness meditation daily.
- Our tone can be more powerful than the words we use.
- Mindfulness practice increases both the activity and size of the prefrontal cortex, which is the area of the brain that regulates our awareness, concentration, decision-making, emotions, and behaviors.

> You can easily access guided meditations on your phone or tablet. Here are a few guided meditation websites, apps, and podcasts to try:
>
> - The Chopra Center (http://chopra.com/)
> - The UCLA Mindful Awareness Research Center (http://hvrd.me/YFbip)
> - Headspace (http://hvrd.me/YFb38)
> - Meditation Oasis (http://www.meditationoasis.com/)

References

Basso, J. C., McHale, A., Ende, V., Oberlin, D. J., & Suzuki, W. A. (2019, January). Brief, daily meditation enhances attention, memory, mood, and emotional regulation in non-experienced meditators. *Behavioural Brain Research, 1*(356), 208–220. https://doi.org/10.1016/j.bbr.2018.08.023

Bru-Luna L. M, Martí-Vilar, M., Merino-Soto, C., Cervera-Santiago, J. L. (2021, December 7). Emotional intelligence measures: A systematic review. *Healthcare, 9*(12), 1696. https://doi.org/10.3390/healthcare9121696

Goleman, D. (2005). *Emotional intelligence: Why it can matter more than IQ*. Random House.

Institute for Mindful Leadership. (n.d.). *Research*. https://instituteformindfulleadership.org/research/

Jefferson Health. (2017). *Professional training*. https://www.jeffersonhealth.org/physicians/professional-education

Kabat-Zinn, J. (1994). *Wherever you go, there you are: Mindfulness meditation in everyday life*. Hachette Books.

Mindful. (2017). *Jon Kabat-Zinn: Defining mindfulness*. https://www.mindful.org/jon-kabat-zinn-defining-mindfulness/

Taren, A. A., Gianaros, P. J., Greco, C. M., Lindsay, E. K., Fairgrieve, A., Brown, K. W., Rosen, R. K., Ferris, J. L., Julson, E., Marsland, A. L., Bursley, J. K., Ramsburg, J., & Creswell, J. D. (2015). Mindfulness meditation training alters stress-related amygdala resting state functional connectivity: A randomized controlled trial. *Social Cognitive and Affective Neuroscience, 10*(12), 1758–1768. https://doi.org/10.1093/scan/nsv066

5
Mind Over Matter

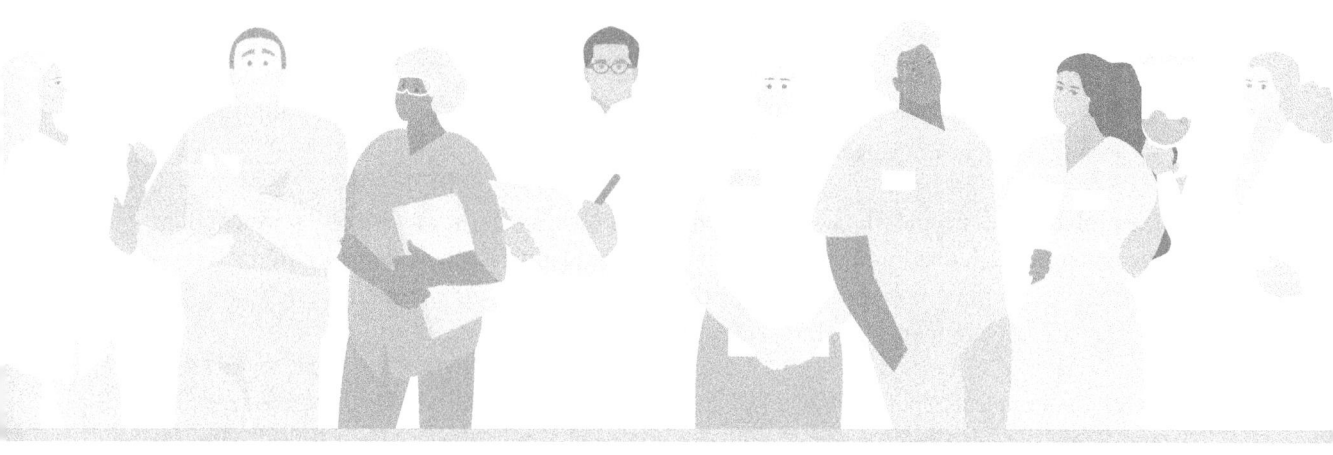

"Your attitude, not your aptitude, will determine your altitude."
–Zig Ziglar

Your ability to use communication to engage, influence, and motivate others is essential for building professional relationships and achieving high-quality patient outcomes. Effective communication lays the foundation for a healthy workplace environment (Babiker et al., 2014; Bru-Luna et al., 2021). Miscommunication in a healthcare environment is both common and costly. Worse, it's a leading cause of mortality and morbidity.

One main reason for ineffective communication is that most people approach situations and conversations with certainty rather than curiosity. We automatically place judgment on someone or something when things go wrong. This is not because we are mean people; it's because of our values, beliefs, and experiences—in other words, our mental model (Dweck, 2006; Gentner & Stevens, 2014).

A *mental model* is a framework we create in our minds to help us interpret or make sense of the world around us. Our mental model guides our perceptions and behaviors and helps us problem-solve and make decisions. Each person's mental model is different.

There are two main types of mental models, or mindsets. One of these is a fixed mindset. Carol Dweck, author of *Mindset: The New Psychology of Success* (2006), observes that people with a fixed mindset assume their intelligence, creativity, and character are set in stone. The other type of mental model is a growth mindset. A growth mindset positions us to be more open-minded and to see things more holistically. Having a growth mindset fosters resilience and enables us to maintain a positive outlook. Those who embody a growth mindset believe that their most fundamental abilities can be developed through hard work, dedication, and perseverance, not just intelligence or talent (Dweck, 2006).

The problem with people who have a fixed mental model is that they filter every problem they encounter through that mindset. As a result, they often fail to accept or consider all the facts—shutting out anything that doesn't mesh with their mindset. As the common proverb says, "If all you have is a hammer, everything looks like a nail."

Here's an example. Suppose a patient tells his nurse that he did not take his prescribed medication. Thanks to her fixed mindset, the nurse immediately concludes that she's dealing with yet another noncompliant patient who thinks he knows best. After further discussion, the patient reveals that he did not take the prescribed medication because he could not afford it and was too embarrassed to tell anyone. Had the nurse maintained a growth mindset, she would have approached the situation with curiosity rather than certainty and would not have been so quick to judge the patient.

Mind Over Matter, or Matter Over Mind?

Recently, researchers conducted an experiment that involved providing students with a nonverbal IQ test that contained several challenging problems. Afterward, the researchers took two different approaches in praising the students for their performance. The researchers told some students, "Wow! You got [X many] problems right! That's a really good score. You must be smart at this!" These were the "ability-praised" students. Other students were "effort-praised." These kids were told, "Wow! You got [X many] problems right! That's a really good score. You must have worked really hard!" In other words, they praised some students for their ability and others for their effort (Dweck, 2006).

In this study, researchers found that effort-praised kids saw the difficulty of the test as an indication that they simply needed to put in more effort to do well, not as a reflection of their intelligence. Moreover, as the questions got more difficult, the effort-praised kids still enjoyed solving the problems. They even said that the more challenging the problems were, the more fun they were to solve. Finally, if they were unable to solve a more difficult problem, they didn't interpret it as a failure on their part. On the other hand, the ability-praised kids had less fun as the questions got harder and felt like failures when they were unable to answer one. Basically, they were discouraged by their success-or-failure attitude and approach.

Ask yourself, do you measure your successes by your abilities or by your effort? To adopt a growth mindset, celebrate your efforts rather than fixating on perfection.

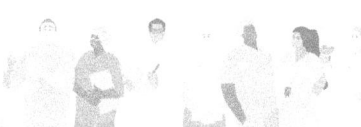

Time to Reflect

Think about a time when you jumped to the wrong conclusion:

- What happened?
- How did you feel after you learned the whole story?
- What did you do about it?
- What would you do differently if it happened again?

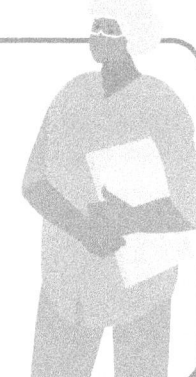

In the Driver's Seat: The Science Behind Communication

Beyond the ideas of a fixed and growth mindset, fields like neuroscience and neuroleadership help us understand the science behind communication. The field of neuroscience focuses on the brain and its impact on behavior and cognitive functions. A subset of neuroscience is an emerging field called *neuroleadership*—a term coined by Dr. David Rock. Neuroleadership applies the concepts of neuroscience to how we interact with each other in the real world.

Neuroleadership provides a deeper understanding of how our brain affects our decisions, workplace relationships, and leadership styles (Rock & Page, 2009). For example, researchers in neuroleadership have found that when people perceive themselves to be socially excluded, it activates their pain receptors. Just think about that: When we exclude people, we cause them to feel *physical pain and suffering*. Research in neuroleadership has also helped us understand why most change initiatives fail—because our brains are hardwired to perceive change as a threat. Indeed, change causes a paroxysm of negative emotions that place the brain and body in fight mode or flight mode (Rock & Page, 2009).

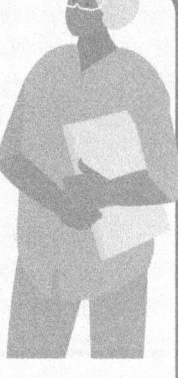

Time to Reflect

- Think about a time when you were excluded from a party, meeting, or special event. How did you feel?
- Have you ever deliberately excluded someone from participating in something that was important to them?
- Have you ever cried so hard that you felt physical pain?
- Have you ever seen someone very upset or cry due to an emotionally charged situation—for example, being newly diagnosed with cancer or having to place a loved one on life support?

The Role of Neurotransmitters

Best-selling author and celebrated TED Talk speaker Simon Sinek (2009) explains how four main neurotransmitters drive our actions and behaviors:

- **Endorphins:** Endorphins are pain-masking chemicals that help us push ourselves through tough circumstances. You see endorphins in action when you witness nurses push through adversity. For example, suppose an influx of patients arrives in the emergency department (ED) all at once. Odds are the nurses in their 10th hour of a 12-hour shift will suddenly have the same amount of energy as they did when they first arrived at work. This is thanks to endorphins.

- **Dopamine:** Dopamine is the goal-achieving chemical. It causes that good feeling we experience when we complete a task. We also experience a dopamine hit when we consume alcohol, nicotine, or drugs; gamble; or even check our email, text messages, or social media. Conversely, when we are prevented from completing a task (or consuming alcohol or nicotine, or gambling, or checking our email or text messages), we often feel frustrated. This is the root of addictive behaviors. Indeed, many people can't get enough of this "feel good" neurochemical. This makes dopamine the most dangerous transmitter of the four listed here.

- **Serotonin:** Serotonin regulates our mood and social behaviors. It's also a key player in our appetite and digestion, sleep, memory, and sexual desire and function. Serotonin surges through our body when we protect and care for others. Simply put, serotonin boosts our confidence and makes us feel happy.

- **Oxytocin:** This neurotransmitter produces the feeling we get from the strong emotional bonds we have with another. In other words, it's the warm feeling we experience when we spend time with someone we enjoy being around, even if we aren't doing anything extraordinary. For example, suppose a nurse is sitting at lunch, sadly reflecting on a recent fetal demise. When a trusted colleague sits next to her, the nurse may suddenly feel comfort and support, even if her colleague hasn't uttered a word. This sense of comfort and support is a product of oxytocin. Note that oxytocin is also responsible for mother-infant bonding—which explains why it is commonly known as the cuddle hormone.

Sinek (2009) further divides these chemicals into two separate categories:

- *Selfish chemicals:* Sinek calls endorphins and dopamine selfish chemicals because it's these chemicals that motivate us to accomplish and achieve things.

- *Selfless chemicals:* Serotonin and oxytocin are called selfless chemicals because they are responsible for cultivating and strengthening the social bonds we have with each other.

> ### Time to Reflect
>
> Consider the following scenario while also thinking about the neurotransmitters discussed in this section and how they might affect how we communicate with each other: A seasoned ED nurse is feverishly caring for an influx of patients with flu-like symptoms. There have also been several callouts during her shift. On top of that, her orientee keeps asking her about things she doesn't think are important just now—what the bathroom code is, who she should contact about her time and attendance, and how holidays are assigned. When the nurse finally snaps at the orientee, the orientee complains. The nurse acknowledges her behavior and apologizes. She then uses this experience as an opportunity to help the orientee deal with the stress of the ED.

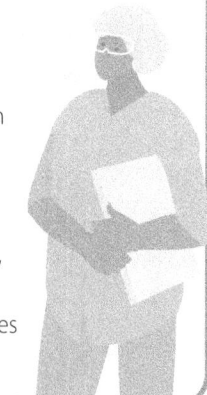

Understanding the Brain-Gut Axis

We often hear people remark that they knew something was going to happen or that they should have trusted their gut. This intuition—often referred to as a gut feeling—is an interesting phenomenon. Most of us do not really know what it is or what to make of it. It is often mistaken for anxiety, doubt, or, in some cases, psychic experiences. One can't help but wonder, does our gut *really* have a sense of its own?

According to psychologist Gerd Gigerenzer, author of *Gut Feelings: The Intelligence of the Unconscious* (2007), the answer is yes. Indeed, Gigerenzer asserts that approximately half of all decisions made at large international companies are made from gut reactions. Moreover, instinct-based choices outperform many choices derived from complex calculations.

Trusting our gut might seem like mystical or even supernatural thinking, but science supports the notion that our gut actually acts as a second brain. This second brain is called the *enteric nervous system* (ENS). The ENS is composed of millions of neurons that line the gastrointestinal tract—more neurons than in the spinal cord or the peripheral nervous system. Neurons in the ENS enable us to "feel" the inner area of our gut. The ENS can identify feelings such as stress or excitement—even if our brain is unable to decipher them. This is because we house more than 90% of our serotonin in our gut. This chemical is transmitted from our gut to our brain (and vice versa) via the vagus nerve (Mayer, 2011).

The ENS receives both conscious and subconscious information from the brain and transmits its own positive or negative responses via somatic markers. These are the sensations we experience when we feel anxious, scared, or excited. Somatic markers are behind that feeling of having butterflies in our stomach, as well as the clenching, tingling, and sweating we often experience—all ways in which we respond physically to real or perceived situations. These symptoms speak volumes about our true feelings—and are often "heard" by others by way of our body language.

Do You Identify as Neurotypical or Neurodivergent?

The terms "neurodivergent" and "neurotypical" are used to describe differences in neurological development and functioning. Here are some key distinctions between neurodivergent and neurotypical individuals:

1. **Neurodevelopment:** Neurodivergent individuals have atypical neurological development compared to the typical or expected developmental patterns observed in neurotypical individuals.

2. **Conditions and traits:** Neurodivergent individuals may have specific conditions or traits that are considered outside the typical range. This can include autism, ADHD, dyslexia, Tourette syndrome, and other neurological differences.

3. **Cognitive and perceptual differences:** Neurodivergent individuals may have unique cognitive and perceptual processing styles. They may excel in certain areas, such as pattern recognition, attention to detail, or divergent thinking. They may also experience challenges in other areas, such as social interactions or sensory processing.

4. **Communication and social interactions:** Neurodivergent individuals may have different communication styles and may struggle with social interactions due to differences in social cognition, understanding nonverbal cues, or social norms. Neurotypical individuals generally conform to the expected social norms and communication patterns.

5. Sensory sensitivities: Neurodivergent individuals may have heightened or reduced sensitivities to sensory stimuli, such as sound, light, touch, or smell. These sensitivities can influence their experiences and preferences.

6. Perspectives and experiences: Neurodivergent individuals often have unique perspectives and experiences shaped by their neurological differences. They may offer alternative viewpoints, approaches, and contributions to society that may differ from the mainstream or neurotypical perspective.

It's important to note that these differences are generalizations, and there is a wide range of diversity within both neurodivergent and neurotypical populations. Each person is unique, and it's essential to recognize and respect individual strengths, challenges, and experiences, irrespective of neurodivergence or neurotypicality.

Are Overthinkers Neurodivergent?

Being neurodivergent does not necessarily mean that an individual is an overthinker. Overthinking is a cognitive tendency or behavior that can be present in individuals regardless of whether they are neurodivergent or neurotypical.

Neurodivergent individuals may have different thinking styles and cognitive processes compared to neurotypical individuals. They may exhibit patterns of thinking that are characteristic of their specific neurodivergent condition. For example, individuals with autism may engage in repetitive thoughts or have intense focus on specific interests. Individuals with ADHD may have racing thoughts or difficulty maintaining attention on a single topic.

While some neurodivergent individuals may experience overthinking as a result of their unique cognitive processes, it is not a defining characteristic of being neurodivergent. Overthinking can occur in individuals across the neurodivergent and neurotypical spectrum and is influenced by various factors such as personality, experiences, and individual traits.

It's important to recognize and address overthinking as a separate aspect that can affect individuals regardless of their neurodivergence or neurotypicality and provide appropriate strategies and support to manage it effectively.

The article "Toward Inclusive Mindsets: Design Opportunities to Represent Neurodivergent Work Experiences to Neurotypical Co-Workers in Virtual Reality" (Lowy et al., 2023) focuses on the use of virtual reality (VR) to promote understanding and inclusivity between neurodivergent individuals and their neurotypical coworkers in the workplace.

The authors highlight the importance of fostering a supportive environment where neurodivergent individuals feel understood and valued. They propose the use of VR as a tool to simulate and represent neurodivergent experiences to neurotypical individuals, enhancing empathy and facilitating better collaboration.

By creating VR simulations that mimic the sensory sensitivities, cognitive differences, and communication challenges faced by neurodivergent individuals, the article suggests that neurotypical coworkers can gain a deeper understanding of their experiences. This increased understanding can help reduce biases, misunderstandings, and stigmatization that may exist in the workplace.

The authors discuss potential design opportunities for VR experiences that aim to represent neurodivergent work experiences. These include creating scenarios that simulate sensory overload, providing interactive elements to demonstrate diverse communication styles, and incorporating decision-making challenges that mimic the cognitive processes of neurodivergent individuals.

The article highlights the potential of VR as a tool to bridge the gap in understanding between neurodivergent and neurotypical individuals, fostering more inclusive work environments. The authors suggest that by designing VR experiences that promote empathy and awareness, organizations can facilitate better collaboration and support for neurodivergent employees.

Overall, the article emphasizes the importance of creating inclusive mindsets and utilizing technology, such as VR, to promote empathy and understanding in the workplace, leading to greater inclusivity and support for neurodivergent individuals.

Your Road Map: Improving Your Mind to Improve Your Outcomes

For many of us, feeling a sense of meaning and value at work is important. This can seem difficult at times, especially when working in the healthcare environment. The ever-changing healthcare landscape places nurses at high risk for burnout, compassion fatigue, and job dissatisfaction. Here are some techniques backed by neuroscience to help you not just survive in challenging times, but thrive:

> If you begin to feel uncomfortable while thinking about a person, issue, or decision, then you have your answer. Your intuition is telling you it's not right. On the contrary, if you feel comfortable, you know it is right.

- **Tune into your intuition.** As you think about people, places, issues, or relationships, your gut will fire a feeling that is associated with those things. When this happens, it's important to become cognizant of what your body is telling you. You can accomplish this by practicing three techniques:
    - **Finding quiet time:** Take a few minutes before you go to sleep, upon waking, and throughout the day to soak in some quiet. You don't necessarily have to block out the world, but you should find somewhere quiet enough for you to hear your own breath. This is a form of mindfulness. For more on mindfulness, refer to Chapter 4.

- **Breathing:** Focus on your breath. Breathe as deeply as you can. Send your breath down toward your stomach and then release it.
- **Listening:** Everyone has a little voice inside that guides them. We just need to listen to it. It's been said that when you quiet the mind, your soul will speak—in other words, the only voice you will hear is your intuition.

Look internally. We often compare ourselves with others. This is a symptom of a fixed mindset. For example, nursing students with a fixed mindset will ask a classmate what they got on an exam and then compare their classmate's grade with their own. In contrast, nursing students with a growth mindset will compare their grade against their own personal trajectory. To stop comparing yourself with others, practice asking yourself, "How am I doing now compared to how I was doing before?" rather than, "How am I doing compared to my colleague?" This shifts your focus from "being good" to "getting better."

Acknowledge and embrace imperfections. If you hide from your weaknesses, you can't overcome them. Instead, adopt a growth mindset and look at challenges as opportunities to learn and grow. You might even go so far as to strike the word "fail" from your vocabulary and replace it with the word "learn." In other words, when errors happen, tell yourself you haven't failed; you've learned.

Value the process. Enjoy the learning process. If it extends beyond the expected time frame, accept it. It takes time to learn, so don't expect to master every topic all at once. Give yourself the gift of time when learning something new. Learning fast isn't the same as learning well—and learning well sometimes requires you to allow time for mistakes. When mistakes happen, don't speak negatively to yourself. Negative thoughts become negative actions.

> Leaders who promote inter-individual comparisons—in other words, "me versus my colleague"—also promote a fixed mindset. In contrast, when leaders promote intra-individual comparisons—think "me now vs. me then"—they promote a growth mindset. This results in increased performance, better learning opportunities, and healthier workplace environments.

Persevere. We all face obstacles from time to time. This can lead to feelings of anger or frustration—which can drive us to quit long before we should. In such situations, don't focus on what has happened *to* you. Instead, focus on what has happened *for* you. In other words, try looking at what your challenges add to you, rather than at what they deplete from you. Looking at obstacles from this upside-down perspective reveals alternative ways to reaching your goal. Don't view setbacks as permanent problems. Instead, see them as temporary situations that you can use to strengthen and empower yourself.

- **Eat right.** Eating healthfully is extremely important for our well-being. Not only does eating healthfully help us improve our physical health (e.g., by losing weight), but it also plays a significant role in brain health. In addition to helping keep your body's immune responses and inflammation under control, your gut produces hormones that enter your brain and influence your cognitive ability. For example, you've probably experienced what I like to call "brain fog" after consuming something unhealthy, like donuts or cake. This occurs because all the sugar in the food alters your gut hormones, which then enter your brain and can cloud your ability to understand and process information. Staying focused on the task at hand and recognizing when you're full also become more challenging. Healthy food choices contain good fats, vitamins, and minerals that provide energy and aid in protecting against brain diseases. Fueling our bodies with whole, nutritious foods benefits our body and our mind.

  > Eat high-quality small snacks, or mini meals, throughout the day. This helps boost your energy and prevent overeating. Also, include healthy, protein-rich foods in your diet. Protein-rich foods help stabilize blood sugar levels, support healthy muscles, and improve the immune system.

- **Exercise.** According to a study conducted at the University of British Columbia, physical exercise can improve memory and executive functioning (Godman, 2014). In addition, a Mayo Clinic study (Sparks, 2013) showed that aging adults who participated in moderate exercise between five and six times a week significantly reduced their risk of experiencing mild cognitive impairments. Adults who routinely exercised early in life reduced their risk even more. Exercise has also been shown to reduce insulin resistance, decrease inflammation, improve our mood and sleep patterns, and reduce stress and anxiety. Even light exercise is better than no activity. Exercise at any time of the day but not at the expense of your sleep.

- **Stick to the same bedtime routine.** Go to sleep and wake up at the same time every day—even on weekends, holidays, and days off. This will reinforce your body's sleep-wake cycle and help you feel less tired throughout the day.

Time to Reflect

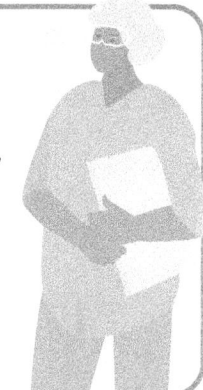

What gives your life meaning? What helps you feel valued at work? What techniques do you use to cultivate and improve what matters to you? To answer these questions, reflect on the following:

- What are your core values and beliefs?
- Who is your idol, and why do you admire this person?
- What do you want your legacy to be?

"Fake It Till You Become It" and the BEST Approach

Dr. Amy Cuddy is a professor and researcher at Harvard Business School whose work incorporates body language, emotional intelligence, and scripting techniques. In a 2012 TED Talk titled "Your Body Language May Shape Who You Are," Cuddy relays a story about suffering a severe head injury in a car accident while earning her undergraduate degree. Doctors told her she would struggle to fully regain her mental capacity.

Due to her head injury, Cuddy struggled to complete her degree. For someone who had always considered herself gifted and intelligent, this was very frightening and upsetting. Fortunately, a close friend gave her some age-old advice: "Fake it till you make it." This advice helped Cuddy reframe her mindset and enabled her to eventually graduate college and even go on to graduate school.

The focus of Cuddy's graduate studies was how nonverbal behaviors and snap judgments affect people from the classroom to the boardroom. Through her research, Cuddy learned a valuable lesson: Her friend's "fake it till you make it" advice was sound but incomplete. A better approach was to "fake it till you *become* it."

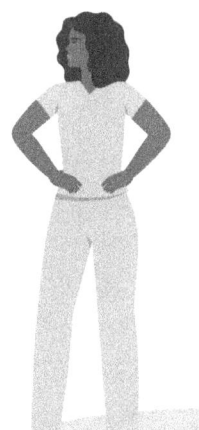

Cuddy has become particularly renowned for her research in something called *power posing* (see Figure 5.1). Power posing pertains to how your body position influences others and even your own brain. Carney and colleagues (2010) assert that simply holding one's body in a wide "high-power" pose for as little as two minutes stimulates higher levels of testosterone (a hormone that triggers feelings of power and dominance) and lower levels of cortisol (the so-called "stress hormone," which can cause impaired immune functioning, hypertension, and memory loss). Indeed, they found that people who held such a pose for two minutes felt increased feelings of power and a greater tolerance for risk.

Figure 5.1 Power posing can influence your mindset to feel more confident.

This research aligns with the BEST approach. According to this approach, we can use our bodies to change our mindset, which in turn can change our actions. In other words:

- **B**ody language: Our body position can change our mindset.
- **E**motional intelligence: Our mindset drives our emotions.
- **S**cripting: Use positive self-talk to believe in yourself.
- **T**ips and techniques: Practice power posing for two minutes.

For example, suppose that after a bad day at work that has left you feeling tired, worn out, and run down, you realize you are scheduled to hold a meeting that evening for a community event. Naturally, this is the last thing you feel like doing. But by applying Cuddy's research and holding your body in a high-power pose for two minutes, you can increase your testosterone and decrease your cortisol. This can give you the extra confidence you need to be successful.

The Drive Home

Let's drive home the key points in this chapter:

- There are many reasons communication is ineffective. One is that most of us approach situations with certainty rather than curiosity.
- What we value, believe in, and experience forms our mental model.
- A mental model is a concept or framework that helps make sense of or interpret the world around us. It helps us understand relationships between things.
- Believing that something can't change in any meaningful way is known as a fixed mindset. A growth mindset allows us to develop a passion for learning rather than craving approval.
- People with a growth mindset have a voracious drive for learning. They constantly seek out input that they can use for learning and constructive action.
- If you begin to feel uncomfortable while thinking about a person, issue, or decision, then you have your answer. Your intuition is telling you something's not right. On the contrary, if you feel comfortable, you can feel confident you're on the right track.
- Four main neurotransmitters drive our actions and behaviors: endorphins, dopamine, serotonin, and oxytocin. Endorphins mask pain, dopamine kicks in when we complete a task or achieve a goal, serotonin boosts our confidence, and oxytocin is the so-called "cuddle hormone."

- In addition to the brain in our skulls, there's a brain in our gut. Choices made from our gut, or our instinct, outperform many that are made through complex calculations.

- Dr. Amy Cuddy's research aligns with the BEST approach. This approach asserts that we can use our bodies to change our mindset and use our mindset to change our behaviors and actions.

- Research indicates that holding one's body in a high-power pose for two minutes can increase testosterone and decrease cortisol, giving us the extra confidence we need to be successful.

References

Babiker, A., El Husseini, M., Al Nemri, A., Al Frayh, A., Al Juryyan, N., Faki, M. O., Assiri, A., Saadi, M. A., Shaikh, F., & Al Zamil, F. (2014). Health care professional development: Working as a team to improve patient care. *Sudanese Journal of Paediatrics, 14*(2), 9–16.

Bru-Luna, L. M., Martí-Vilar, M., Merino-Soto, C., & Cervera-Santiago, J. L. (2021, December 7). Emotional intelligence measures: A systematic review. *Healthcare, 9*(12), 1696. https://doi.org/10.3390/healthcare9121696

Carney, D. R., Cuddy, A. J., & Yap, A. J. (2010). Power posing: Brief nonverbal displays affect neuroendocrine levels and risk tolerance. *Psychological Science, 21*(10), 1363–1368. https://doi.org/10.1177/0956797610383437

Cuddy, A. (2012). *Your body language may shape who you are* [YouTube video]. https://www.youtube.com/watch?v=Ks-_Mh1QhMc

Dweck, C. S. (2006). *Mindset: The new psychology of success.* Random House.

Gentner, D., & Stevens, A. L. (2014). *Mental models.* Psychology Press.

Gigerenzer, G. (2007). *Gut feelings: The intelligence of the unconscious.* Allen Lane.

Godman, H. (2014, April 9). *Regular exercise changes the brain to improve memory, thinking skills.* Harvard Health Publishing. https://www.health.harvard.edu/blog/regular-exercise-changes-brain-improve-memory-thinking-skills-201404097110

Lowy, R., Gao, L., Hall, K., & Kim, J. G. (2023, April). Toward inclusive mindsets: Design opportunities to represent neurodivergent work experiences to neurotypical co-workers in virtual reality. *Journal of Workplace Inclusivity, 8*(2), 123–145. https://doi.org/10.1145/3544548.3581399

Mayer, E. A. (2011). Gut feelings: The emerging biology of gut–brain communication. *Nature Reviews Neuroscience, 12*(8), 453–466. https://doi.org/10.1038/nrn3071

Rock, D., & Page, L. J. (2009). *Coaching with the brain in mind: Foundations for practice.* John Wiley & Sons.

Sinek, S. (2009). *Start with why: How great leaders inspire everyone to take action.* Portfolio.

Sparks, D. (2013, May 14). *Regular physical exercise has powerful impact on brain health.* Mayo Clinic. https://newsnetwork.mayoclinic.org/discussion/tuesday-q-a-regular-physical-exercise-has-powerful-effect-on-brain-health/

6

Impromptu Scripting, Phrasing, and Acronyms

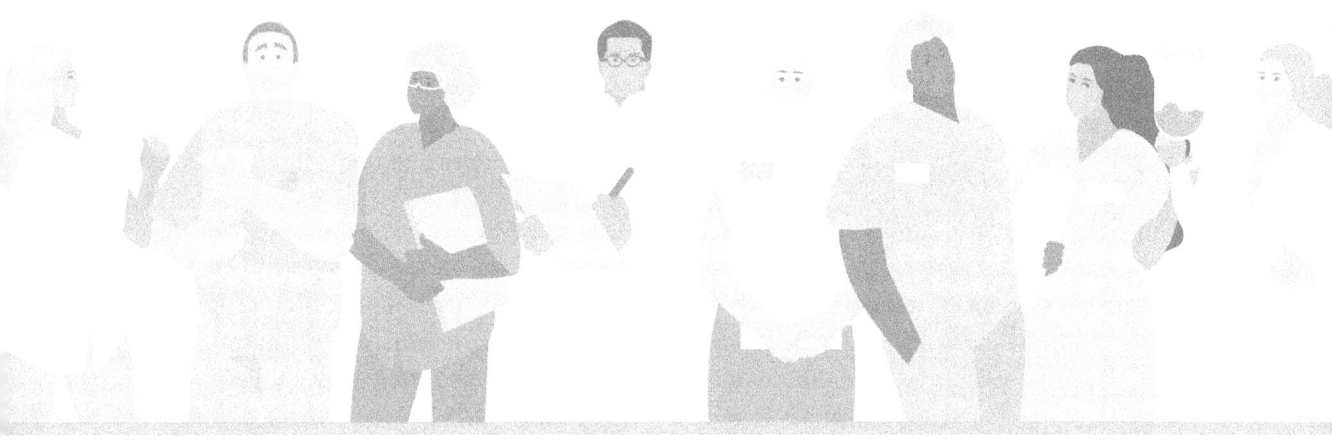

"It is better to keep your mouth closed and let people think you are a fool than to open it and remove all doubt."
–Mark Twain

To script or not to script: In healthcare, that is the question.

According to Merriam-Webster (n.d.), to *script* is to plan how something will happen or be done. Scripts are very useful since they are simple, easy-to-remember phrases that provide the language that goes into a specific conversation. Scripts might include ice breakers, conversation starters, and key speaking points. Scripting enables us to naturally deliver thoughtful and appropriate phrases or responses. It also helps us deliver a consistent, service-oriented response. Finally, it can help us change topics or redirect or even end a conversation.

Those opposed to scripting argue that it seems staged or robotic. That's a fair criticism. To deliver a script with authenticity, one must have ownership of the script and truly believe it. Otherwise, it sounds rehearsed. I tend to disagree, however. After all, think about how many times you use scripting without even realizing it. For example, when you run into an old friend by surprise, odds are you automatically resort to scripted phrases like the following:

- "Hello! How are you?"
- "Hey, how have you been?"
- "Oh my goodness, what have you been up to?"
- "Wow! It's been so long!"

You probably also use certain "scripted" nonverbal gestures, such as smiling, raising your hands palms up with your elbows at your waist in a welcoming gesture, or placing your hands on your cheeks or over your mouth to convey that you're speechless.

Now imagine you had similar automatic scripted responses when faced with a less desirable situation. Wouldn't that make your life easier? I have found it invaluable to have several hard-wired scripts available, depending on the situation. The idea is not to memorize these scripts; rather, it's to use them as a guide when responding to various emotionally charged situations. At the same time, you need not reinvent the wheel each time you use these scripts, either. Instead, you can build upon what has worked before and adapt them for new situations. This chapter introduces you to several impromptu scripts and provides several acronyms to make these scripts easier to remember.

In the Driver's Seat: Using Impromptu Scripts

Have you ever felt like a deer in headlights during a difficult conversation with a patient, colleague, or executive—unsure of what to say and what *not* to say? Many of us have. Being in a highly emotional or serious situation increases your stress levels, triggering a strong emotional response that decreases your ability to think logically, respond rationally, and find just the right word or phrase (Goleman, 1998). This is why using scripts in your everyday conversations can be very advantageous. Table 6.1 shows some examples of useful scripts for complex leadership and management situations.

Table 6.1 Using Scripting to Address Challenging Situations

WHAT TO SAY	WHAT NOT TO SAY	RATIONALE
"I would like to think this over first. I'll have some time to discuss this later."	"Well, you may have time to discuss this, but I don't."	This script gives you time to cool off, calm down, or just think about the problem and devise a solution.
"I'd really like to help you with your patient, but I'm working with Mrs. Smith right now. I just can't ignore my current responsibilities."	"No."	Just saying "no" sounds cold and standoffish. Briefly explaining why you can't do something helps the other person understand the barriers you face.
"I'm just finishing something up right now. Can I stop by your unit when I'm finished?"	"I don't have time to talk to you."	Telling someone you don't have time to talk to them—whether in person or on the phone—is just plain rude. Instead, explain why you are unable to talk just now and suggest a better time for you.
"I'm prioritizing my time on _____ right now."	"That's not my job."	When approached with tasks that are not within your primary role (and when you don't have time to help out), reinforce your primary responsibilities.
WHEN UNCERTAIN OR CONFUSED		
WHAT TO SAY	**WHAT NOT TO SAY**	**RATIONALE**
"Could you clarify your comment about _____?"	"This may sound dumb, but…"	Be clear and respectful but not self-deprecating when asking for clarification.

continues

Table 6.1 Using Scripting to Address Challenging Situations (cont.)

WHEN UNCERTAIN OR CONFUSED		
WHAT TO SAY	**WHAT NOT TO SAY**	**RATIONALE**
"I will find out," or, "I will look into this."	"I don't know."	Promising to investigate a matter is a savvy way of stating that you don't have an answer yet, but you will help find one.
"What I hear you saying is _____."	"Aha."	You'll likely get more details when you paraphrase what you heard.
WHEN FEELING CONFIDENT OR APPRECIATIVE		
WHAT TO SAY	**WHAT NOT TO SAY**	**RATIONALE**
"Thank you."	"OK."	Saying "thank you" is common courtesy. Whether given in private or in public, a sincere "thanks" fosters goodwill.
"I'm on it."	"I guess I'll have to do it."	When you say, "I'm on it," what you're *really* saying is, "Relax. Don't worry about a thing. I'll see to it personally." That response can defuse just about any situation.
"My pleasure," or, "I'm happy to help."	"No problem."	It's better to say that you are happy to help or assist than to suggest their request might have been a "problem" for you.

Your Road Map: Acronyms and Emotional Intelligence

According to The Joint Commission (2023), "Failures in communications, teamwork and consistently following policies were the leading causes for reported sentinel events. Most reported sentinel events occurred in a hospital (88%). Of all the sentinel events, 20% were associated with patient death, 44% with severe temporary harm and 13% with unexpected additional care/extended stay" (para. 3). Fortunately, scripting can help with this. This section covers useful acronyms for scripts and the application of emotional intelligence in scripting.

Useful Acronyms for Scripts

There are several acronyms to help nurses remember various scripts. One of these is SBAR. Using the SBAR acronym—which has been endorsed by the American Nurses Association—

helps healthcare providers ensure they are communicating effectively during patient handoffs to provide all critical information needed. SBAR stands for (Kaiser Permanente of Colorado, 2004, para. 2):

- **Situation:** Provide a concise statement of the problem or situation.
- **Background:** Briefly convey pertinent information about the situation.
- **Assessment:** Provide an analysis and state what options have been considered (in other words, what you found and think).
- **Recommendation:** Request an action or provide a recommendation.

Piggybacking off the SBAR concept, you can also use acronyms to help elicit feedback from others. One such acronym is 3WITH. The purpose of 3WITH is to remind you to ask open-ended questions. 3WITH stands for the following (see Figure 6.1):

- **3W:** This refers to the three key words that start with W: what, why, and where. For example, "What did you do?" "Why did that happen?" or "Where did this stem from?"
- **I:** This stands for "in what way."
- **T:** This stands for "tell me more."
- **H:** This stands for three key words that start with H: heard, help, and how. For example, "I heard you say…," "Help me understand…," and "How can I help you?"

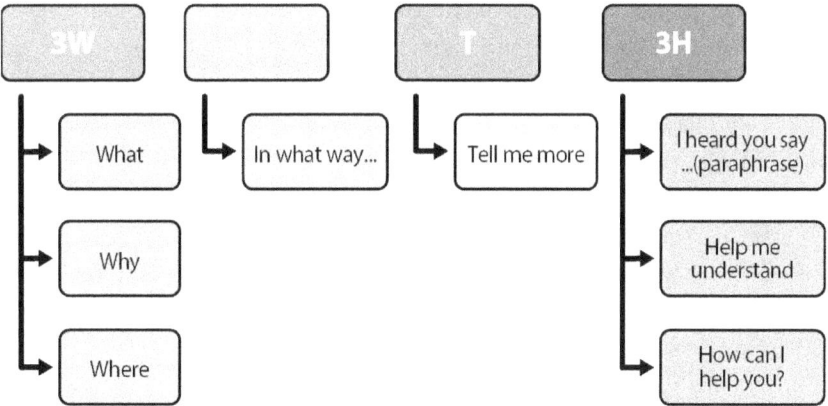

Figure 6.1 The 3WITH method.

> Asking open-ended questions elicits better responses. Open-ended questions remove bias and can help you gauge whether someone's body gestures match their words. For example, if you ask someone how he is feeling, and he says "Fine" but drops his head wearily, then you know there's a disconnect, which may require further probing on your part. Finally, open-ended questions can help you confirm (or not) what you perceived and understood.

Script 6.1 shows how you can incorporate the 3WITH acronym when working with a patient you feel is being disrespectful. Notice how easily the patient's demands could have been interpreted as disrespectful. Continually asking open-ended questions reveals what's *really* going on with the patient.

Applying Emotional Intelligence to Scripting

Acronyms and scripting techniques are only as useful in conversations as your level of emotional intelligence (EI) and emotional competence (EC). In other words, you may have hardwired yourself to formulate open-ended questions, but if you ask these questions with no regard to your emotions or those of the person with whom you are speaking, it will be useless if emotions are running high. Indeed, you are more likely to receive *no* response if you or the person you're speaking to is emotionally unstable. This section reviews key components of EI and EC and outlines some scripting techniques and acronyms you can use to tap into them.

Self-Awareness

According to Showry and Manasa (2014), "Self-awareness in general denotes subjective and accurate knowledge of one's inner self, e.g., mental state, emotions, sensations, beliefs, desires and personality. It comprises beliefs, intentions and attitudes about oneself based on experiences in life" (p. 16). Being self-aware means having a clear picture of your strengths and weaknesses. This helps us adopt a growth mindset and be more accepting of ourselves and others (Heckemann et al., 2015).

Self-awareness helps keep you in check regarding how your emotions affect you and others (Goleman, 2005). When it comes to communicating, being self-aware means knowing your emotions and examining your tone when speaking and listening to others. To improve your self-awareness and communication, try using the LEARN acronym:

- **Listen:** What is your inner voice telling you? Is this positive or negative self-talk?
- **Empathize:** How did your actions or behavior affect others?
- **Ask:** Use active listening skills and ask clarifying questions to ensure your communications are effective and maintain a growth mindset.

- **Recognize** your emotions and feelings: Name them to tame them.
- **Notice** how others receive your emotions and feelings: Do your colleagues perceive you as being poised and in control of your emotions or behaving unprofessionally?

Self-Regulation

Recall from Chapter 3 that the part of your brain called the *amygdala* dictates how you respond to emotionally charged situations, flooding your body with stress hormones when it perceives a threat. This is often called an *amygdala hijack*. The following statements may indicate an amygdala hijacking:

- "What was I thinking? I'm such an idiot!"
- "I'll never get this project finished."
- "That's it. I can't take it anymore!"
- "This place is just toxic and chaotic."
- "No one around here cares about me."
- "If they don't want to listen to me, then—oh well!"
- "I'll never be nice to him again."

When you make statements like these, you are not taking responsibility for the situation. Rather, you are putting the responsibility for the situation on other people. To correct your thought process, you must take responsibility for the situation. This involves identifying your emotions and taking control of them—in other words, self-regulating.

Having high EI and EC enables you to self-regulate to remain poised and professional in the face of an amygdala hijacking. Self-regulation keeps us in tune with and in control of our emotions. Nurses who can self-regulate rarely attack others, make hasty or emotionally based decisions, stereotype people, or show disrespect. To become aware of your emotions and how you regulate them, ask yourself the following types of 3WITH open-ended questions:

- How and what am I feeling?
- How long have I felt this way?
- What is my body doing in response to feelings—for example, am I clenching my teeth, feeling tired, or experiencing a headache or stomachache?

Asking yourself these simple questions enables you to obtain a rational understanding of your emotions and to gain better control of them. You are thinking things through before responding rather than just blurting out the first thing you think of thanks to your amygdala!

SCRIPT 6.1

What to say when…

YOU THINK A PATIENT ISN'T BEING RESPECTFUL TO YOU (USING THE 3WITH ACRONYM).

T
Time and place to talk

Find an appropriate time and place to address the issue with the patient. Ensure privacy and a calm environment where you can have a conversation without distractions.

> Excuse me, Joe (patient). As the doctor just explained, you are going to be discharged home today, so please help me understand why you are asking me to brush your teeth and wash you today?

E
Explain and explore perspectives

Clearly and assertively express your concern about the patient's disrespectful behavior. Be specific about the actions or words that were disrespectful and how they have affected you or others involved in their care.

Example: Disrespectful

> Well, I have been brushing my teeth every day—along with washing myself and feeding myself. Don't you nurses take care of patients anymore? I have Medicare insurance, so you're getting paid to do your job.

> (Ask open-ended questions to unveil what is not being said). Joe, it is important that you take care of yourself when you can. Why do you think nurses need to do basic hygiene care if a patient is more than capable?

> I thought nurses were supposed to take care of sick people. You haven't done any of this for me. I'm once again left to do everything myself. You nurses these days aren't as good as they were years ago. A good nurse then would have attended to me more.

> Nurses do care for the sick and assist patients when needed. Tell me more, Joe. I'm not sure I understand why you're so upset.

> Look, I just wanted my ol' teeth brushed. (Silence) Ah geez, OK well, my brother was in this very same hospital and had his teeth brushed, and they washed them. He said how comforting it was, and I'm getting the raw end of the stick. He just said to me this morning that his car accident years ago was much more serious than why I am here. But, of course, he always has one on me.

L
Listen to their perspective

Allow the patient to express their concerns or frustrations that may have led to their disrespectful behavior. Practice active listening and empathize with their situation, while still maintaining firm boundaries regarding respectful communication.

Example: Sympathetic

> I'm sorry you are feeling this way. It sounds like your brother couldn't do basic care for himself when he was hospitalized. Fortunately, you are strong enough to be independent. Tell me how you feel about your independence.

> Hey, you know, I have to be independent. I'm all I got. The wife passed years ago, and the kids live across the country. I have friends and neighbors, but it's not the same as when my wife was here.

> I see. So in your situation, independence isn't always what you want. Please correct me, but what I'm hearing is that you may have wanted me to brush your teeth just so you could take a little break from doing everything all by yourself?

L
Leverage shared values and lead the conversation forward

Remind the patient of the shared goal of providing quality care and achieving positive outcomes. Emphasize the importance of mutual respect in fostering a productive and supportive patient-provider relationship.

Example: Apologetic

> Well, every day I have to do everything alone, and I guess I let my brother's comments make me feel even more alone. (Pause) Hey, thank you for talking to me. Getting old isn't easy.

> I'm happy I could be here for you and talk this through. What else can I do for you, Joe? I have the time.

> Brush my teeth? (Patient laughs and affirms his comment was meant to make the nurse smile.)

On a related note, of course, we have all said or done something less than desirable and punished ourselves afterward with negative thoughts and self-talk. Fortunately, you can learn to reframe this negative self-talk into positive self-talk to keep yourself focused and on track. Alternatives to the negative self-talk phrases might include the following:

- "I made an honest mistake. This is frustrating, but I can undoubtedly fix it."
- "I need to refocus on the priorities and ask for help."
- "I need to take a pause so my frustration doesn't prevent me from doing a good job."
- "My ideas aren't always the ones chosen. Maybe I should get feedback on this one."
- "Let me make sure I fully understand the initiative. What else can I do to help get us there?"
- "He may be someone who doesn't want a friendly relationship with me, and that's OK."

Time to Reflect

What does it mean to be proactive rather than reactive? The word *reactive* suggests you let events set the agenda. In other words, you react to events rather than guiding them. To be proactive means you anticipate what the future might be and act accordingly—*before* it happens.

Consider the following reactive and proactive statements. What are some other examples of these types of statements?

REACTIVE STATEMENTS	PROACTIVE STATEMENTS
"Well, I did what I could…"	"I will search for and consider alternatives."
"It's just who I am."	"I can make a different choice."
"She makes me so mad."	"I can control my feelings."
"I have to do that."	"I will choose an appropriate retort."
"I can't _____."	"I prefer to _____."

Responding to Bad News

Suppose you were asked to work on a very important project for the Magnet® application with an elite group of nurses. A month later—after countless hours of blood, sweat, and tears—your group submits this assignment to the chief nursing officer (CNO). The CNO reviews your work and sends it back to the group with more corrections than you had expected. You can't help but notice there wasn't even one positive comment made! How do you react when you receive this news?

- **Feeling:** Do you feel angry? Scared? Embarrassed?
- **Thinking:** What is your initial thought? How does this mesh with how you are feeling?
- **Physical reaction:** Is your heart racing? Are you breathing more quickly than normal? Did you lose your appetite?
- **Behavior:** Did you punch a wall? Put your head down? Cry?

Suppose you immediately speak to the CNO about her feedback. If you let your emotions run the show, the conversation will likely go like this:

> **Nurse (feeling like a victim):** "But Janet, we spent a lot of time on this!"
>
> **CNO:** "This is not the level of work I was expecting from this team."
>
> **Nurse (feeling angry, confused, and upset):** "I beg to differ. You don't understand how much effort we put into this. This is crazy! I just can't believe this. I don't know what will make you happy!"

A much better approach to this conversation—which, again, occurred immediately after you received the CNO's message—would be to remain calm, ask the CNO to repeat her comments, and then state verbally that you understand them. You may discover in this exchange that the criticism is based on a misunderstanding or is a result of the CNO having a different perspective—in which case it should be reasonably straightforward to iron it out.

In a more complicated situation, you should schedule an "offline" meeting to discuss the criticism. For example, you might say the following:

> **Nurse (taking a deep breath and remaining calm):** "It is important to our team that we are successful on this project. I would like clarification on a few of your comments. When is a good time to set up a meeting?"

Then, when the meeting occurs, you should calmly rephrase the CNO's complaints in your own words to make sure you understand them. For example, you could start with a phrase like, "So, what you're saying is…," or, "To clarify…." As you speak, you should use a nonaggressive tone and make eye contact with the CNO. The goal is to remove the focus from any personality clash and place it directly on substantive disputes.

This approach also works if the CNO's assessment of the project is unreasonable, as it may shine a harsh light on the initial critique. You must be very careful, however, to stay factual. Avoid the temptation to exaggerate. If the CNO claims your work was mediocre, don't say, "So what you're saying is that our work is not good enough for the Magnet document." Overstating the case in this manner will cause you to come off as defensive rather than as someone who is truly looking to get to the bottom of the problem. A rational response is the best antidote to unfair criticism. Often, it wins out—if the people involved are open and willing to finding the best course.

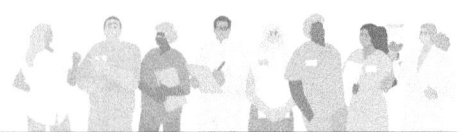

Motivation

Strong leaders lead by example to motivate others. They also use high-impact motivational language in their communications. Table 6.2 contains examples of high-impact motivational words and how to use them.

Table 6.2 High-Impact Motivational Words and How to Use Them

HIGH-IMPACT MOTIVATIONAL WORD	EXAMPLE OF USE
Positive	"I am positive about our choice."
Fabulous	"That is a fabulous idea."
Absolutely	"I absolutely agree…."
Certainly	"I can certainly assist you…."
Wonderful	"That is a wonderful alternative…."
Fantastic	"What a fantastic solution."
Completely	"I completely agree with your concern."
Indeed	"Indeed, this will help…."
Unquestionably	"That is unquestionably the solution."
Definitely	"I am definitely interested."

Empathy

Nurses must have empathy to deliver excellent care. This requires nurses to be socially aware to gauge how patients, families, and colleagues are feeling. This is no small task considering that people rarely tell us how they really feel about something.

Think about the standard greeting in the workplace: "Hello. How are you today?" Regardless of how they are actually feeling, receivers typically respond with something along the lines of, "I'm good, thanks!"

To become aware of another person's *true* feelings, nurses must ask open-ended questions. The responses to these open-ended questions can help nurses read between the lines of what the receiver is saying to gauge how the person is really feeling. Here are a few examples:

- "How can I help you?"
- "Tell me more about that."
- "What type of resolution are you hoping for?"

There are also some standard phrases you can use to improve your social awareness and increase your level of empathy. These are shown in Table 6.3.

Table 6.3 Phrases for Social Awareness and Empathy

PHRASE	EXAMPLE	EXPLANATION
"I imagine…"	"I imagine you'll be sitting up by the end of the day!"	This tells your listener that you're just exercising your imagination and not trying to be judgmental.
"That reminds me…"	"You saying you went down to the lab reminds me—did you know there is a new process for obtaining blood gases?"	This transition-type phrase helps to connect topics. It's helpful when you want to change the topic but keep the conversation flowing—or even to completely redirect the conversation.
"Let's pretend…"	"I see you are in a lot of pain. While your medication is beginning to work, let's pretend we're on a sunny beach on a beautiful day!" "Let's pretend our boss says no to the proposal. We can always remind him of what happened the last time he said no!"	This phrase invites others to join you in leaving reality for a brief time. This is also a wonderful way to gain permission to play devil's advocate or show the opposing side to an argument without appearing threatening or judgmental.
"I would like to…"	"Although I don't work in the labor and delivery unit, I would like to!"	This phrase helps you show interest in something.

When using these types of questions and phrases, you must consider your tone. Your tone should be empathetic. In other words, what you say and how you say it should match up.

The Impact of Past Experiences on One's Level of Empathy

There is conflicting research on whether past experiences improve one's level of empathy. According to Lombardo and Eyre (2011), nurses who have experienced emotional extremes themselves are more likely to show empathy for others because they understand how they feel. On the other hand, Ruttan and colleagues (2015) found that a person who has experienced an adversity similar to someone else often evaluates the other person's experience more harshly.

Relationship Management

Nurses with strong social skills know how to manage their relationships with patients, families, and colleagues. One technique they use to achieve this is to avoid undermining someone else's thoughts and feelings. This is incredibly important. It is OK to disagree, but it is not OK to be disrespectful or judgmental when you do. In other words, you should steer clear of statements like the following:

- "I understand how you're feeling, but I don't think you understand."
- "I can understand why you feel that way, but you're wrong."
- "I appreciate what you are telling me, but I think you are really off base."

> Sometimes you can't get around using the word **"but."** But (see?) if you can, you should. Often, saying "but" discounts everything you said before it. For example, consider this compliment: "I like your scrub top, but I like the one you wore yesterday." This statement could be interpreted to mean you actually *don't* like the top the person is wearing today. In this case, it would be best to replace the word "but" with **"and"** or **"so"**—as in, "I like your scrub top, and I like the one you wore yesterday, too!" This keeps the conversation positive.

When you find yourself disagreeing with someone, don't try to convince them your view is correct. Instead, try to understand why they feel the way they do. It could be they perceive the issue or situation differently—perhaps in some way you haven't considered. In other words, treat the other person's feelings as information you need to process. Here are some phrases you might use to learn more and to maintain the flow of communication:

- "Tell me why you feel that way."
- "What aspect of the project/idea/decision makes you feel that way?"
- "What is it that you need?"
- "I understand that you feel this way. How can we gain your support in the decision?"
- "I can see that you are very uncomfortable with the decision. Tell me more."
- "I know you are hesitant and that you only want us to be successful."
- "I hear the concern in what you are saying, and I appreciate it."
- "I haven't experienced what you are feeling. I imagine it is not easy."

In addition to demonstrating that you're considering the other person's needs and helping them achieve their goal, these statements also validate and empower them—truly a win-win situation! Table 6.4 contains a few more helpful phrases to help you manage relationships and keep communication flowing.

Table 6.4 Phrases for Relationship Management

PHRASE	EXAMPLE	EXPLANATION
"…just kidding!"	"This is my first day in the OR, and you are my very first patient ever…just kidding! I've been here for 15 years and assisted in hundreds of these surgeries. I can assure you that you are in good hands!"	This is the best way to backtrack out of something that the listener may have perceived as inappropriate (which you can gauge by their body language). The key is to say this phrase before the listener reacts verbally.
"I can relate to…"	"I can't imagine how you felt while awaiting your sister's diagnosis, but I can relate to being scared about things, like when we thought my brother would have to have his leg amputated."	Sometimes the best way to relate to someone is to tell a story of a time you faced a situation similar to theirs to show you have commonalities and understand how they may be feeling.
"I don't know too much about that, but I'm guessing it's similar to…"	"I don't know too much about that since I never worked in the cath lab, but I'm guessing it's similar to my unit in terms of its unique challenges!"	This is the perfect transition-type phrase to keep a conversation going even if you have no knowledge of the topic. It's OK to admit your ignorance; just use this phrase to fill in the gap.

Another important aspect of relationship management is conflict management. Conflict management involves a complex skill set. Your ability to manage conflict is invaluable and will help you become a better nurse, coworker, and leader.

When resolving conflict, many of us obey the Golden Rule—treating others as we wish to be treated. Business experts Alessandra and O'Connor (1996) suggest a different approach: treating others as *they* wish to be treated (not as *we* wish to be treated). They call this the Platinum Rule. Remember: We all have different needs, wants, and desires. We need to think about how we can best serve others in their way, not ours. That's what the Platinum Rule is about.

Of course, this begs the question: How can we know what other people want? I suggest considering the four social styles discussed in Chapter 1. For example, suppose you have an amiable social style and tend to focus on emotions and feelings. If you were resolving a conflict with someone who had a similar social style, then you could reasonably treat them as you wish to be treated. Someone with a driving social style, however, would not react well to this approach (Merrill & Reid, 1981). This type of person will generally prefer a direct, quick, and specific resolution.

Other ways to improve your conflict-management skills include the following:

- Setting ground rules for the conversation—for example, saying there will be no interruptions allowed
- Asking open-ended questions to reveal the genesis of the conflict
- Allowing people to share their feelings and concerns without judgment

Pulling It All Together With the CAR Framework

Recall from prior chapters how the BEST framework incorporates body language, emotional intelligence, and scripting techniques for more effective communications. Recall, too, that you can apply the CAR framework within the BEST framework. In this case, you can do this to think through the specifics of how, why, where, and when you will engage others in conversations.

- **Consideration:** As discussed in Chapter 1, the C in the CAR framework reminds you to consider the Five Rights of Communication Safety. This helps you ensure you're speaking to the right person, at the right place, at the right time, with the right emotions in check, and with the right intent. This will depend on your EI and EC, as well as your ability to interpret body language. Conducting conversations at the right time can be further assessed with regard to our emotional sensitivity, as shown in Figure 6.2.

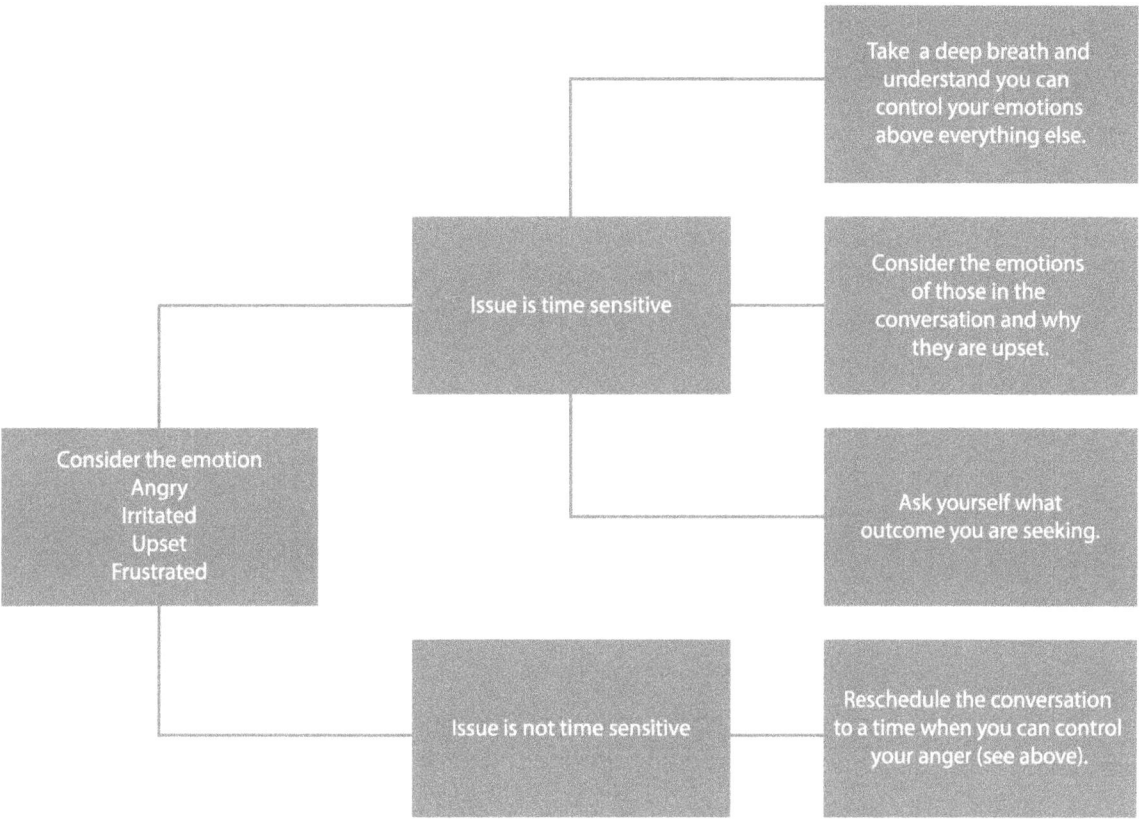

Figure 6.2 Decision tree for time-sensitive decisions.

- **Action or call to action:** The action or call to action enables you to plan the conversation—including what specific acronyms or scripting techniques you will use. If you need to deliver the same message to two different people, you may need to communicate it differently each time due to varying social styles.

- **Return on investment:** Identify your desired return on investment (ROI) before having a conversation. This involves pinpointing why you're having the conversation to begin with and determining what a successful conversation would look like to you. With this information in hand, you can determine which acronyms and scripting techniques to use.

> While we're talking about investment, suppose your emotions are running high. If you allow these emotions to drive your behavior, you are at risk of having a poor outcome. Is this worth investing in?

The Drive Home

Let's drive home the key points in this chapter:

- Hardwiring a few positive and motivating scripts can help you deter future amygdala hijackings, which results in improved communication and relationship management.

- Weaving scripting into open-ended questions helps you remember what words to use, remove bias, and gauge whether someone's body language matches the words they use.

- 3WITH stands for what, why, and where; "in what way"; "tell me more"; and heard, help, and how.

- To resolve conflict, we must consider how best to serve others in *their* way, not ours.

- The CAR framework calls on you to:

  - Consider whether you are speaking to the right person, at the right place, at the right time, with the right emotions in check (EI and body language), and with the right intent.

  - Identify the correct action or call to action based on the other person's social style. One size doesn't always fit all.

  - Identify the desired ROI—that is, the outcome you seek in having the conversation. To prevent your investment from ending up in the red, avoid lashing out, and reframe negative self-talk to be positive so it leads to a productive action.

References

Alessandra, T., & O'Connor, M. J. (1996). *The Platinum Rule: Discover the four basic business personalities—and how they can lead you to success*. Grand Central Publishing.

Goleman, D. (1998). *Working with emotional intelligence*. Bloomsbury Publishing.

Goleman, D. (2005). *Emotional intelligence: Why it can matter more than IQ*. Random House.

Heckemann, B., Schols, J. M., & Halfens, R. J. (2015). A reflective framework to foster emotionally intelligent leadership in nursing. *Journal of Nursing Management, 23*(6), 744–753. https://doi.org/10.1111/jonm.12204

The Joint Commission. (2023.) *New sentinel event data available for 2022*. https://www.jointcommission.org/resources/news-and-multimedia/newsletters/newsletters/joint-commission-online/april-5-2023/new-sentinel-event-data-available-for-2022/

Kaiser Permanente of Colorado. (2004). *SBAR technique for communication: A situational briefing model*. Agency for Healthcare Research and Quality. https://www.scribd.com/document/391825094/SBARReport-NurseStudent

Lombardo, B., & Eyre, C. (2011). Compassion fatigue: A nurse's primer. *Online Journal of Issues in Nursing, 16*(1). https://doi.org/10.3912/OJIN.Vol16No01Man03

Merriam-Webster. (n.d.). Script. In *Merriam-Webster.com dictionary*. https://www.merriam-webster.com/dictionary/script

Merrill, D. W., & Reid, R. H. (1981). *Personal styles and effective performance*. CRC Press.

Ruttan, R. L., McDonnell, M. H., & Nordgren, L. F. (2015). Having "been there" doesn't mean I care: When prior experience reduces compassion for emotional distress. *Journal of Personality and Social Psychology, 108*(4), 610–622. https://doi.org/10.1037/pspi0000012

Showry, M., & Manasa, K. V. L. (2014). Self-awareness: Key to effective leadership. *The IUP Journal of Soft Skills, 8*(1), 15–26.

7

Interprofessional Coaching Conversations

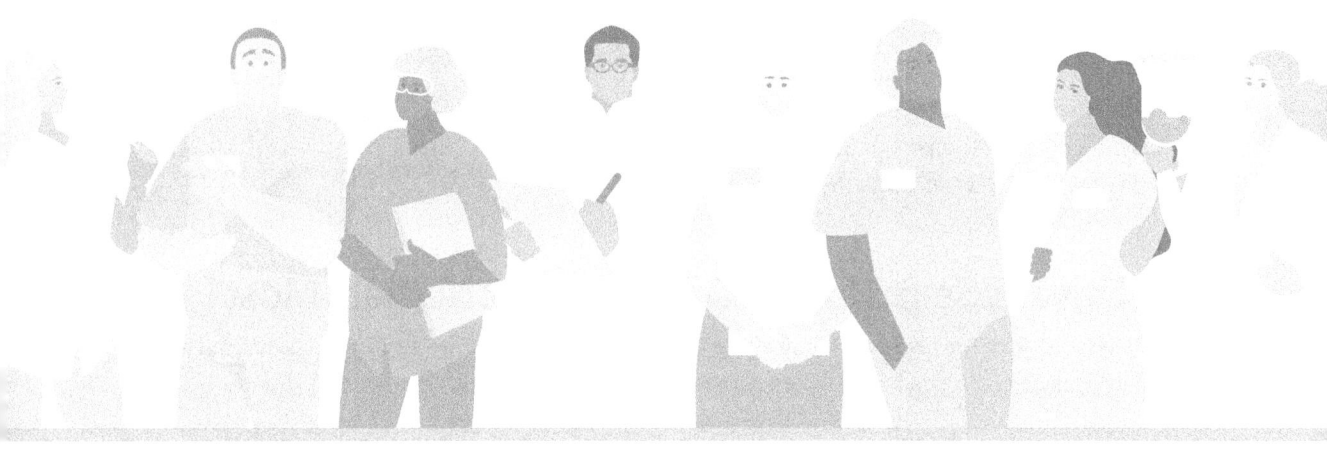

"If your actions inspire others to dream more, learn more, do more, and become more, you are a leader."
–John Quincy Adams

Instead of using common descriptors like "courageous conversations" or "difficult conversations" in the title for this chapter, I purposefully used the phrase "coaching conversations" to help reframe the negative connotations associated with those terms. Examples of interprofessional coaching conversations might include:

- Talking to a coworker about a problem she's having that is affecting your work
- Giving your nurse manager feedback when she's doing something that's demotivating you
- Providing corrective criticism to a colleague
- Talking to a colleague, doctor, or patient who is not keeping up her end of a bargain
- Confronting a coworker or colleague about disrespectful behavior, such as discrimination
- Pointing out someone's shortcomings that are affecting patient care (e.g., noticing that a colleague didn't wash her hands)

These types of conversations are just plain hard—especially when emotions are high or the conversation involves someone you sincerely like (or dislike). Not surprisingly, most people tend to avoid these conversations completely, hoping the situation will miraculously improve. A better alternative is to learn the skills needed to have effective coaching conversations and then facilitate the dialogue with grace and finesse. That's the focus of this chapter.

> Interprofessional coaching conversations can help others better contribute toward a shared goal, enhance their competence and commitment, and improve relationships.

In the Driver's Seat: How to Discuss What Matters Most

When faced with the prospect of engaging in a hard-to-have conversation, it can be helpful to have scripts in place, such as the ones outlined in Scripts 7.1 and 7.2.

The primary purpose of a having a hard-to-have conversation is not to persuade or get one over on the other person. It is to explain what you see, why you see it that way, and how you feel about it, and to come to a resolution—and for the other person to do the same. You simply can't move the conversation in a more positive direction until both people feel they have been heard and understood. Each person involved in any situation has a different story about what happened; your job is not to judge who's right and who's wrong but to manage the situation to achieve a better outcome.

> If you find that others don't listen to you, consider whether you need to spend more time listening to them. Or consider whether when you "try" to listen, your body language indicates otherwise.

It follows, then, that a real conversation is an interactive process in which you are constantly listening. Listening shifts the goal of the conversation from trying to persuade someone to actually learning from them. As a bonus, when you listen, you increase the likelihood that the other person will listen to you.

Formal and Informal Nurse Leadership Training

Regardless of your title, you are a leader. Indeed, all nurses are leaders—whether formal or informal. Therefore, when issues arise, it is your professional responsibility to adopt an approach that is solution-oriented, not problem-oriented. Nurses who constantly run to those in formal leadership roles to seek solutions to their problems miss a big opportunity to be viewed as leaders themselves.

The quality of your leadership skills is reflected in the quality of your interprofessional conversations—which has larger ramifications. For example, if a nurse manager does not conduct effective conversations—offering feedback and coaching—the whole organization is affected. Similarly, when frontline nurse leaders communicate poorly to colleagues or patients, the result will be friction, pushback, and eventually the breakdown of the team—not to mention a waste of time and energy.

One way for healthcare organizations to facilitate a solution-oriented approach is to offer leadership training for all nurses. Leadership training is essential for improved patient outcomes. It also facilitates strong employee engagement (Kelly et al., 2014). Sadly, most healthcare organizations either don't provide leadership training for nurses (Curtis et al., 2011; Sherman et al., 2007; Shirey, 2006; Swearingen, 2009) or don't allow nurses the time to attend the training (Kivland & King, 2015).

Nurse leaders in particular need leadership training to help develop strong professional relationships with members of their teams. This becomes even more urgent when one considers that, according to Gallup, the number-one reason Americans switch jobs is their poor relationship with their manager or boss (Lavoie-Tremblay et al., 2016).

Another core competency taught in leadership training is human resources management. More specifically, leaders are taught about the importance of employee rounding. Employee rounding provides an opportunity for leaders to identify gaps in processes or systems, establish relationships, show appreciation, and, ultimately, build trust (Cochrane, 2017; Schuller et al., 2015). And rounding with departmental managers or directors strengthens interdepartmental relationships. (See Appendix A, "Sample Rounding Template," for more information.)

> Regardless of whether we are formal or informal nurse leaders, improving our leadership skills is a shared responsibility. Refining our leadership skills is truly a journey to excellence.

SCRIPT 7.1

What to say when…

YOU WANT TO ASK YOUR MANAGER TO STOP MICROMANAGING YOU.

T
Time and place to talk

Find an appropriate time and place to discuss the issue with your nurse manager or supervisor. Choose a calm and private setting where you can have an uninterrupted conversation.

Example: Nurse Manager

> Excuse me, Judy. I would like to speak with you about our mutual involvement in [insert name of project]. I appreciate that you asked me to take the lead on this. I'm just hoping you can explain why I need to obtain your approval before moving onto the next level.

E
Explain and explore perspectives

Clearly and assertively express your concerns about being micromanaged. Provide specific examples of instances where you felt micromanaged and explain how it has affected your work and productivity.

Example A: Understanding

> I didn't realize I was doing this. You're right, I don't need to approve this at every level.

> Great, thank you. I'll still keep you abreast of my progress, though.

Example B: Defensive

> Well, I just want to make sure you're on the right track.

> I appreciate your concern. But I'm worried you might not be comfortable with my judgment.

L
Listen to their perspective

Allow your nurse manager or supervisor to share their perspective on the situation. Listen actively and try to understand their reasons or concerns behind the micromanagement. Keep an open mind while still asserting your need for autonomy and trust.

Example A: Understanding

> How should we proceed?

> Moving forward, I'd like to send you a summary of how I will complete the next section of the project, and you can give me feedback. Does that sound reasonable?

Example B: Defensive

> *I never said I was uncomfortable with your judgment. Like I said, I just want to make sure you're on target. This is a big proposal.*

I was hoping I could be more instrumental in the decision-making process. I would like to complete [insert task] and then gain your insight. Is it acceptable from this point forward that I meet with you [insert time] and at that time you can provide further guidance, instead of me submitting this every day for your approval?

L
Leverage shared values and lead the conversation forward

Remind your nurse manager or supervisor about the shared goals and objectives of your role. Emphasize the importance of trust, empowerment, and autonomy in achieving those goals. Highlight how micromanagement can impact your motivation and hinder your ability to contribute effectively.

Example A: Receptive

> *Great, that sounds reasonable.*

Thank you for your support. I really appreciate it. I'll send you a meeting request today.

Example B: Unreceptive

> *I need to think about this.*

I respect that. Is there anything else I can do in the meantime?

(If the manager is unreceptive, ask more open-ended questions to understand why they need to be so involved in every aspect of the initiative(s) at hand. The consequences may be that you will need to continue working in this way.)

SCRIPT 7.2

What to say when…

YOU FEEL A COLLEAGUE ISN'T RESPECTING DIVERSITY.

T
Time and place to talk

Choose an appropriate time and place to address the issue. Find a moment when you and your colleague can have a private conversation without distractions.

Example: Coworker

> Owen, I was told you didn't think Shweta (coworker) could handle the project since she is from India.

E
Explain and explore perspectives

Clearly and assertively explain that you have noticed instances where your colleague has not been respecting diversity. Be specific about the behaviors or comments that you find concerning.

Example A: Denial

> No, I didn't.

> I'm glad this source was incorrect because that was a very offensive comment.

Example B: Excuse

> Oh, come on, it was funny.

> I'm sure that was your intent, but it was offensive, not funny.

Example C: Doubling Down

> Well, it's true!

> Your personal feelings have nothing to do with her performance. Your accusation is inappropriate.

L
Listen to their perspective

Allow your colleague to share their perspective and understand their reasoning behind their actions or comments. Practice active listening and try to grasp their viewpoint while still maintaining your commitment to promoting diversity and inclusion.

Example A: Denial

> *No, I didn't.*

> *It's a shame people feel the need to undermine others because of varied backgrounds. I hope you would join me in confronting staff who do this and even report it.*

Example B: Excuse

> *I was just joking.*

> *Can you share with me why I thought your comment was so inappropriate? (Teach back.)*

L
Leverage shared values and lead the conversation forward

Example C: Apologizes

> *You're right, I did say that. I'm sorry.*

> *If I ever hear such a comment again, I will report you on that occurrence and provide documentation on this prior occurrence and this conversation as well.*

Remind your colleague of the shared goals and values related to diversity and inclusion within your workplace. Emphasize the importance of respect and acceptance in creating a harmonious and productive work environment.

At this point, either take further action or move forward. Either way, you showed Owen his accusations are not tolerated.

Replacing Certainty With Curiosity

Chapter 5 discusses improving communication skills by moving from a place of certainty to a place of curiosity in your conversations. For example, when someone thinks differently from you, try moving from a thought process that results in questions like:

- "How can they think that?"
- "How can they be so unreasonable?"

to a more curious thought process, such as:

- "I wonder what information they have that I don't."
- "How do they see things so that it makes sense to them?"

Developing a curious mindset isn't easy. The first step is to realize that understanding someone doesn't mean you are agreeing with them. You're simply respecting their views and admitting that they may have different information about and a different interpretation of the situation at hand. Simply acknowledging this can earn you a lot of respect. For example, you might say something like, "Now that we understand each other, what would you like to do to solve this problem?" This doesn't mean that you are giving in to someone; it simply opens the door for finding resolution.

This approach also helps to separate blame from contributions in conversations. Blame is about judging others and draws on negativity. When you ask, "Who is to blame?" you are essentially asking three negative questions:

- Who is responsible for the problem?
- Were they incompetent, unreasonable, or unethical?
- What punitive action is now warranted for their actions?

> Although being punitive may be appropriate in some bureaucratic situations, it is often just a substitute for figuring out the root cause of the problem—that is, what really happened and why.

Identifying contributions is different—and more positive. This involves asking questions like, "How have we each contributed to this condition?" and, "What can we do to move forward?"

Time to Reflect

Some people look to blame others (or even themselves) when things don't go right. The next time you find yourself stuck in blame, ask yourself the following questions:

- What feelings am I not expressing?
- Has the other person acknowledged my feelings?

Alternatively, try using a role-reversal approach. Ask yourself:

- What would the other person say *I'm* contributing to this negative situation?

Work through your feelings and any distortions or gaps in your perceptions. Then share your feelings by saying something like, "Although this was probably not your intention, I felt uncomfortable when I heard you say _____." This shows you are taking responsibility for your contribution.

You should also describe how your contribution has affected the situation. For example, you could say something like, "I feel there are a few things that I've done [or not done] that have made this situation worse. I'd like to discuss this with you."

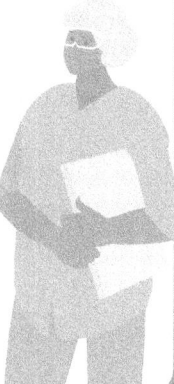

Coaching Conversations: The Six Rules of Etiquette

- Don't judge, blame, or fault others.
- What you would like for yourself, give to another.
- Change your perspective to change your perception.
- It's not what you say but how you say it.
- Perception is someone's reality until proven otherwise.
- Feelings aren't right or wrong—they simply *are*.

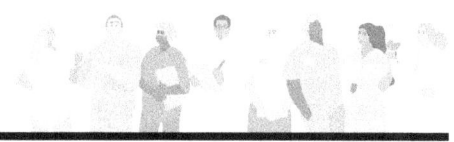

Framing Coaching Conversations

Coaching conversations take a direct approach. And just like a story or movie, coaching conversations have a beginning, a middle, and an end. The beginning provides the structure and the intent, or purpose, of the conversation. The middle is when experiences, perceptions, and feelings are shared. At the end, all parties should reach an agreement that satisfies their mutual interests.

The beginning of the conversation should be relatively brief. You're simply introducing (or even reintroducing) the issue. The middle of the conversation takes the most time. This is the part where you listen to each other and gain an understanding of each other's issues and concerns. During the end of the conversation, you simply set expectations moving forward and wrap up the conversation. It is very important to have structure in a coaching conversation.

Throughout the conversation, ask open-ended questions. Here are some examples:

- What could we do differently to achieve our desired result?
- How can we meet the needs of the operation *and* the team/patient/family?
- What have we not yet tried? What else could be done?
- What specifically is working for us right now? How can we build on that?
- How can I assist others to help me? What can others do to help me?
- How am I currently viewing this situation? Is that the most useful perspective?
- What can I do to make the greatest difference at this point in time?

Many of my colleagues observe that starting these types of conversations is the most difficult step. They ask, "How do I even bring up an uncomfortable topic?" I usually explain that if they feel a little apprehensive, chances are high the other person does, too. Here are some examples of good ways to initiate a coaching conversation:

- "I want to suggest a way to discuss _____ that provides us both time to think and respond to what's being said. I'm open to the possibility that I've either missed something or in some way contributed to this, so I'd like to hear your reactions to what I'm going to share, and I'd also appreciate your perspective."
- "Here's how I thought we could begin: I'll start by describing my perspective, such as what I remember about what happened, and then you can share your reaction to this with me."

- "It's important to me that I share how I'm feeling about this situation and the impact it's had on me, and I'd like to hear your thoughts on that. Then I'd like to explore ways we could ensure that when we work together in the future, we work effectively."

The bottom line: You need to keep sight of your goal. Go into coaching conversations with a clear and realistic preferred outcome. Remember: Winning is not a realistic outcome because the other person is unlikely to accept the outcome of losing. If you prepare for the conversation, follow a solid conversational structure, and remain in a curious and resourceful emotional state, then the likelihood of reaching a desired outcome for all parties is high.

> **Coaching discussions aren't confined to vertical interactions, such as those between nurse leaders and staff members. They can also occur horizontally, involving exchanges between colleagues on the same level.**

Time to Reflect

One of the best ways to prepare for hard-to-have coaching conversations is to ask yourself the following questions and reflect on your responses. Through this process, you can explore possible issues before they catch you by surprise.

- What makes you nervous about this conversation?
- What are you most worried about?
- What personal issues come to mind as you anticipate this conversation?
- What hot topics come to mind around this conversation?
- Think of a time you handled a difficult conversation well. Then think of a time you handled a difficult conversation poorly. How might your attitude, affect, or behavior have played a role in those circumstances?
- What would you most like to happen in this upcoming conversation?
- What can you do to increase the likelihood of this happening?
- What might you do that would impede it?

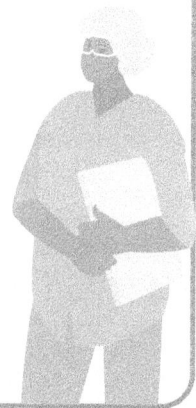

Dealing With Common Emotions During a Coaching Conversation

Suppose you've finally found the strength to initiate a coaching conversation. Just as you begin to talk about your intent for the conversation, the other person immediately grows angry and defensive and begins to cry.

The fact is, high emotions are contagious. To protect yourself, you have to get vaccinated. This is not to say you should become completely immune to other people's emotions. You can sympathize. But don't fall victim to having your emotions hijacked. Remain calm and composed in the face of the other person's emotion. Stay matter of fact, without judgment or disapproval. This can help to de-escalate the emotion and enable the other person to regain some sense of control.

Here are a few scripting suggestions to deal with common emotional responses:

- **Crying:** "I can see you are upset. I will give you a moment to compose yourself before we continue."
- **Anger:** "I understand that this situation is difficult and frustrating. If you need a minute, please take it. We're going to work through this issue to resolution, so I need you to remain calm."
- **Blaming:** "I understand that there are other people involved, but this conversation is about you and me. Those other employees will be dealt with in the same respectful manner that I am dealing with you right now."
- **Bringing up past complaints:** "I understand that you have other concerns, and we can schedule time to talk about them later. Right now, I want to focus on _____."

Overcoming Conversational Traps

Over the years, I've observed several conversational traps. One common one is what I call a *conversation sandwich*. In a conversation sandwich, the conversation starts and ends with something positive, while the "meat" of the conversation—the hard part—is sandwiched in between.

Here's an example: A colleague of mine called one of her direct reports into her office to discuss tardiness. My office was adjacent to hers, and I couldn't help but overhear the conversation. When the employee walked into my colleague's office, my colleague began the conversation by saying, "Oh, I love your shoes today. You look so nice!" Then she dove into the "meat" of the sandwich, saying, "I am really worried about your tardiness. What is up with you lately? I need you to get your act together!" Then, without even giving the employee a minute to speak, my colleague concluded the conversation with, "Oh, and hey, by the way, thanks again for running that blood down to the lab for me."

Don't get me wrong: I am completely in favor of positive feedback. But positive conversations are for reinforcing positive behaviors and should not be woven into hard-to-have coaching conversations. These conversations need to be direct and focused. Otherwise, it's just too confusing.

Another conversational trap occurs when conversations become so heated there is absolutely no room for anything positive to emerge from them. These conversations are like a battle. Everyone's adrenaline is on overdrive. Finding a resolution is impossible; all that happens is yet more issues are uncovered. In the fog of this type of conversation, it's easy to forget that everyone involved is dealing with high emotions and that you don't have access to anyone's intentions but your own. If you find yourself stuck in this mire, try saying, "I'm realizing as we talk that I don't fully understand how you see this problem." This respectful observation is a very powerful way to redirect the conversation back to its original purpose.

> Being clear and direct is far more respectful than attempting to soften a hard-to-have conversation.

Walking Away

If you find yourself in a heated conversation and you can't redirect it to become more positive, it's OK to walk away. First, though, do the following:

- **Explain why you are walking away.** Otherwise, you may give the other person the idea that they must be right because you have nothing else to say.
- **Explain what you need for resolution and which needs haven't been met.** This gives the other person clear insight as to what your expectations are.
- **Be willing to accept the consequences.** Walking away might result in a cooling-off period…or further escalation.

Then there are *sly foxes*. These are people who fall into the conversational trap of using words that are general, undermining, toxic, extreme, condescending, or made up. For example, consider the following conversation between Dr. Kelly, a CCU Nursing Director, and Dr. Smith, a CCU Medical Director at the same hospital. In this conversation, Dr. Smith plays the sly fox, speaking antagonistically toward Dr. Kelly. (His sly fox behaviors are indicated in brackets.) This puts Dr. Kelly on the defensive.

> **Dr. Smith:** "Look Dr. Kelly, everybody knows [general] that this process-improvement project is supposed to be finished by the end of June. The only reason we are not going to meet the deadline is because of your slow [toxic] nursing department."

Dr. Kelly: "My nursing team is not slow! We have a much better record than other teams around here. And the reason we can't hit the deadline is because we don't have the resources."

Dr. Smith: "Somehow, I knew you were going to use that as an excuse [undermining Dr. Kelly]. I don't know if this is true [undermining himself], but I heard that the executive team gave you three extra people to work on this part of the project [made up]!"

Dr. Kelly: "That's not true. I needed people with specific skill sets, and we rotated the nursing team members for this."

Dr. Smith: "The fact is that you think you can get anything you want around here for this little part of a big project and still be able to fall back on excuses why it's not done on time [condescending]."

Dr. Kelly: "I cannot believe this! I feel that I am being marginalized here."

Dr. Smith: "It is absolutely clear [extreme] that the reason your team is failing [toxic] is that they lack a strong nursing leader [undermining]!"

Rather than playing the sly fox, it's far better to play the cool cat. Cool cats stick to the facts, acknowledge their feelings and the feelings of those around them, and respectfully seek resolution. To become a cool cat, Dr. Smith should use less extreme language and stick to facts, not his assumptions. Here are a few suggestions he (and you) could use:

- **Don't generalize by saying "everybody" this or "everyone" that.** Instead, speak from your own observation and leave out information that is merely hearsay. For example: "As you know, we were given a deadline of June 30. As I look at our progress to date, I'm worried we will not make the deadline."
- **Stick to the facts.** Don't assume your personal views or perceptions are facts. When you do share your views or perceptions, use language like:
    - "As I understand…"
    - "There have been some developments that I believe you might not be aware of…."
    - "In my opinion…"
- **Don't undermine yourself.** If you're not sure something is true, don't say it. If you do know, indicate how you know—for example, by saying, "I have heard from two people that…." Or phrase it as a question: "Can you tell me more about…?"

- **Don't undermine others.** To understand their position, ask thought-provoking questions such as:

    "Help me understand why you chose X instead of Y."

    "How did you conclude that…?"

    "What can we do to solve this?"

- **Don't be dramatic or condescending.** Instead of saying, "The fact is [insert story or perception]," or, "It is clear that…," simply state, "From what you said, my understanding is…."

Coaching Conversation Do's and Don'ts

Do

- Ask open-ended questions using the 3WITH method, such as:

    "What would that look like?"

    "What information might you have that I don't?"

    "How do you see it differently?"

    "Tell me more."

    "Help me understand better."

- Paraphrase what you've heard to clarify what you are learning.

Don't

- Disguise a claim as a question.
- Use questions to cross-examine.
- Use negative body language.

Taking Time to Reflect

After a coaching conversation takes place, the speaker has an opportunity to reflect on what worked well and on how she could have improved the conversation. Similarly, the listener can reflect on the feedback received. For example, suppose an upset patient speaks to the unit's nurse manager because her nurse has not responded to her numerous call-button requests in a timely manner. The nurse manager then speaks to the nurse in question to obtain her perspective. First, though, the nurse manager takes a moment to prepare how she will deliver a coaching conversation to the nurse should the situation escalate. And if the situation does escalate, the nurse manager will take a moment to reflect on what worked well in the conversation and what she could have improved upon.

Your Road Map: Applying the BEST Approach in Coaching Conversations

Suppose you are the nurse manager (NM) of a primary care pediatric practice. On a dreary day in mid-November, you take on a full patient assignment because you have three registered nurse (RN) callouts, and you're also trying to run the flu clinic and meet payroll deadlines. Out of nowhere, the Medical Practice Director, Dr. Todd, commands you to have an immediate conversation with one of your RNs, named Susie.

"Susie seems to be experiencing many difficulties in obtaining proper head measurements," Dr. Todd, none too pleased, informs you. "She consistently makes errors in obtaining and documenting head circumference." Dr. Todd, now irate, continues: "How could you possibly allow someone so incompetent to work at this practice?" Before you can respond, he jabs a finger in your direction, barks, "Fix it…*or else*," and storms off.

After this exchange, you're left feeling a mix of emotions: angry because Dr. Todd didn't acknowledge how much you have on your plate right now, embarrassed because you hadn't noticed Susie's skills were that bad, and apprehensive because you find disciplining staff to be the most awkward part of your roles and responsibilities. You are simply not a fan of conflict.

Understandably, you (the NM) feel like you need to "fix" this problem immediately. The result is the following exchange:

> **NM (with arms crossed and an accusatory tone):** "Susie, our Medical Director informed me that you are not obtaining head circumferences correctly."
>
> **Susie (with arms crossed and rolling her eyes):** "What is he talking about? I'm taking the measurements correctly!"
>
> **NM (with arms crossed, hand on chin, and a perplexed facial expression):** "Dr. Todd says otherwise. I have a full patient load today and a million other things to do. I really don't need this right now."

> Planning and self-reflection are at the core of the ROI piece of the CAR framework—both before the conversation and after. Before the conversation, the ROI piece reminds you to explore your intent for the conversation. Afterward, you can reflect on how the conversation went—what went well, what could have gone better, and what you might have done differently.

Susie (with hands on both hips and weight shifted to the right hip in a defensive stance): "I don't know what to tell you. I know what I'm doing, and he never said anything to me."

NM (sensing Susie's defensiveness, backing down, and using a skeptical tone as she walks away): "OK, well, just make sure you double-check yourself, especially around Dr. Todd."

Needless to say, this was not an effective conversation. A better tactic would have been to use the BEST approach to ensure you used the right words and body language. The next section takes a closer look at how you can use the BEST approach in coaching conversations by incorporating the CAR acronym and the TELL acronym.

Pulling It All Together With the CAR Acronym

Let's apply the CAR framework within the BEST approach to make a hard-to-have conversation a little easier on you. Recall that the CAR acronym is the framework of the BEST approach and stands for consideration, action or call to action, and return on investment (ROI).

When preparing for a coaching conversation in a scenario like the one described in the preceding section, consider the Five Rights of Communication Safety:

- **Right person:** Are you sure the RN named by the doctor is truly the person at fault? Also, who else might need to know about the conversation before it takes place?

- **Right place:** Here's a good rule of thumb: Coach in private, commend in public. With this rule in mind, you should plan for this coaching conversation to take place in a private setting.

- **Right time:** Is now an appropriate time for the conversation? In other words, will immediately taking the RN aside disrupt patient flow? Also, is the issue current or one that occurred some time ago?

- **Right emotion:** Are your emotions or that of the RN too high to conduct the conversation just now? Remember: Elevated emotions decrease your chances of an effective conversation. Also, have you thought through the problem enough to articulate it well? Finally, consider what internal or external factors might be causing the RN to behave as she does.

- **Right intent/ROI:** What outcome do you seek? Is the conversation meant to be educational, disciplinary, informational, or something else? Is the outcome you seek one the RN can reasonably achieve? Are you willing to experience the emotions that may arise because of this conversation? Also consider how important it really is to bring up this problem, what would happen if you didn't have this conversation, and who or what else this conversation might affect.

As for your action or action plan: Consider how you will structure this coaching conversation. In this case, I suggest you use the TELL approach (described in the next section).

Finally, to identify the ROI, you need to not only pinpoint the outcome you seek but also note how this outcome will resolve the situation. In other words, are you looking for the RN to just agree with you? Or are you looking for her not to agree with you but to improve her performance? (If it's the latter, then you need to be prepared to help her develop an action plan.)

Pulling It All Together With the TELL Acronym

Now that you've reviewed the CAR framework, it's time to apply the TELL acronym to learn how to make critical conversations like the one between you as the NM and Susie more effective:

- **T – Time and place to talk:** Choose an appropriate time and place for the conversation where both parties can have privacy, minimal interruptions, and sufficient time to discuss the matter thoroughly.

- **E – Explain and explore perspectives:** Explain why the issue you've raised is a problem and extract the other person's story of the account. When doing so, avoid statements that start with "You make me feel…" in favor of statements that begin with "I feel." The goal is to keep the conversation factual and calm by *describing* your feelings rather than acting them out. Be specific: Say, "I'm angry," "I'm worried," or "I'm annoyed."

- **L – Listen to their perspective:** Allow the other person to share how they see the situation. Take the time to pause and listen. When appropriate, show the other person what good performance looks like—in terms of the work (e.g., demonstrating to Susie how to properly take head measurements) *and* during the conversation. Regarding the latter, avoid blame, judgment, and condescension when articulating the desired new behavior. The key is to ask for a positive change rather than a negative one. In other words, try saying something like, "Please try to be more open to the opinions of others by asking open-ended questions," rather than, "Stop being so critical!"

- **L – Leverage shared values and lead the conversation forward:** Be clear about any consequences the person will face if they fail to improve performance. If the consequence will be disciplinary in nature, be prepared to carry it out. Otherwise, you'll lose credibility. Also, if you have developed a performance improvement plan, you can share that now. For example, you could say, "If you will work with me on this, then I am confident that both you and the team will benefit. If not, I will be forced to start formal disciplinary action according to our human resources policy."

As you employ the TELL acronym, maintain control over your body language and work to interpret the body language exhibited by the other person. Tables 7.1 through 7.4 walk you through using the TELL approach to conduct a coaching conversation complete with body language cues, again using the Susie example.

Table 7.1 Using the Time and Place to Talk Component of the TELL Acronym

BODY LANGUAGE (NM)	BODY LANGUAGE (RN)	EI/EC (NM)	EI/EC (RN)	SCRIPTING TECHNIQUES	CONVERSATION
NM maintains eye contact. NM is relaxed. NM places arm out to direct RN into an office.	RN maintains eye contact. RN grabs a pad and pen. RN runs hands through hair while walking to the office.	NM remains in control of emotions.	RN feels a little uneasy. RN questions what this meeting is about.	NM is considerate of RN's time.	NM: "Susie, do you have a few minutes to talk?" RN: "Yes."
NM folds hands lightly on table. NM turns midsection toward RN.	RN crosses arms. RN wraps ankles around chair legs.	NM remains in control of emotions.	RN feels more uncomfortable and defensive.	NM is straightforward, to the point.	NM: "Susie, it has come to my attention that you're not obtaining head circumferences correctly."

Table 7.2 Using the Explain and Explore Perspectives Component of the TELL Acronym

BODY LANGUAGE (NM)	BODY LANGUAGE (RN)	EI/EC (NM)	EI/EC (RN)	SCRIPTING TECHNIQUES	CONVERSATION
NM maintains eye contact. NM leans in toward RN. NM's belly button faces RN. NM steeples hands on table.	RN maintains eye contact. RN crosses arms. RN wraps ankles around chair legs.	NM remains in control of emotions.	RN feels more uncomfortable due to the accusation but appreciates recognition of her hard work.	NM remains positive and validates RN's contributions to the office.	NM: "Susie, you have been a great asset to us for the past three months of your employment. You come to work on time, you're happy, and you work hard. I was quite shocked to hear from a colleague that you are having difficulty with this task. Can you share with me your thoughts on this?"
NM folds hands lightly on table. NM turns midsection toward RN.	RN cups neck with hands. RN leans toward NM. RN wraps ankles around chair legs.	NM remains in control of emotions. NM observes that RN's body language indicates she is upset.	RN feels worried. RN does not feel angry.		RN: "I am shocked, too. No one ever said this to me before. Who said this? Am I being fired?"
NM opens palms and places them face up, revealing openness. NM turns midsection toward RN.	RN cups neck with hands. RN leans toward NM. RN wraps ankles around chair legs. RN looks to the left often.	NM remains in control of her emotions and senses RN is upset.	RN feels worried. RN does not feel angry. RN begins to feel inquisitive. RN recalls how she usually performs head measurements.	NM is motivating and positive. NM acknowledges RN's feelings by stating she isn't being fired.	NM: "I didn't receive permission to share who said this, but it is more important that we identify where the mistake is, if any, and how we can fix it. You are not being fired. I know it is not your intention to take inaccurate measurements. Let's work together on an action plan."

Table 7.3 Using the Listen to Their Perspective Component of the TELL Acronym

BODY LANGUAGE (NM)	BODY LANGUAGE (RN)	EI/EC (NM)	EI/EC (RN)	SCRIPTING TECHNIQUES	CONVERSATION
NM maintains eye contact. NM maintains open arms. NM stands tall.	RN maintains eye contact. RN initially crosses arms. As teaching begins, RN leans toward NM. RN's pelvic area directly faces tape measure held by NM.	NM remains confident, approachable, and in control of emotions.	RN feels uncomfortable. RN becomes interested in NM's measuring technique.	NM is straightforward in her conversation and teaching. NM is not punitive.	NM: "I want to perform the head circumference in front of you on the next patient. Let's go bring the patient back to the exam room." [NM preps patient and performs head circumference measurement. The patient leaves.] NM: "I measure heads on the eyebrows and at the top of the occipital bone, not above the eyebrow and at the largest spot on the back of the head." RN: "I see I was doing it incorrectly. I'll do the next measurement as you watch me to ensure I am measuring correctly moving forward."

Table 7.4 Using the Leverage Shared Values and Lead the Conversation Forward Component of the TELL Acronym

BODY LANGUAGE (NM)	BODY LANGUAGE (RN)	EI/EC (NM)	EI/EC (RN)	SCRIPTING TECHNIQUES	CONVERSATION
NM maintains eye contact. NM maintains open arms. NM stands tall.	RN maintains eye contact. RN initially crosses arms. As teaching begins, RN leans toward NM. RN's pelvic area directly faces tape measure held by NM.	NM remains confident, approachable, and in control of emotions.	RN feels uncomfortable. RN becomes interested in NM's measuring technique.	NM is straightforward in her conversation and teaching. NM is not punitive.	NM: "Susie, I will watch how you perform the next head circumference measurement and will provide feedback. I will also watch the next three measurements. Please know, this is considered a coaching session, based on our performance management policy. I strongly encourage you to ask me for help if you are uncertain of anything. I will be periodically checking you to ensure this practice is sustained. If you do not continue in this manner, we will move toward disciplinary action. Can you share with me what you understood from our conversation, and do you have any further questions?" RN: [Correctly paraphrases her understanding of the problem and the resolution.]

The Drive Home

Let's drive home the key points in this chapter:

- Each person involved in any situation has a different story about what happened. Your goal is not to judge who's right and wrong but to manage the situation for a better outcome.

- After someone tells you her point of view, paraphrase or summarize it back to her. This not only ensures you understand her position but also tells her that you were listening and you care.

- Anger, tears, and denial are all possible outcomes of a coaching conversation. Although you can't control how the other person will react, you can anticipate these reactions and be emotionally prepared to deal with them.

- Stay consistent in your delivery of hard-to-have conversations. Don't deliver a conversation sandwich—starting and ending with something positive, with the "meat" of the discussion in between.

- The best feedback is straightforward and simple.

- The CAR approach is a framework for coaching conversations and can help infuse the BEST approach into the conversation.

- The TELL acronym is a reminder to consider the time, place, and intent of the conversation; explain and explore perspectives; listen to the other person's perspective; and ultimately leverage the conversation for a mutually agreeable outcome.

References

Cochrane, B. S. (2017). Leaders go first: Creating and sustaining a culture of high performance. *Healthcare Management Forum, 30*(5), 229–232. https://doi.org/10.1177/0840470417718195

Curtis, E. A., Sheerin, F. K., & de Vries, J. D. (2011). Developing leadership in nursing: The impact of education and training. *British Journal of Nursing, 20*(6), 344–352. https://doi.org/10.12968/bjon.2011.20.6.344

Kelly, L. A., Wicker, T. L., & Gerkin, R. D. (2014). The relationship of training and education to leadership practices in frontline nurse leaders. *Journal of Nursing Administration, 44*(3), 158-163. https://doi.org/10.1097/NNA.0000000000000044

Kivland, C., & King, N. (2015). *Six reasons why leadership training fails.* Executive Learning Exchange. https://www.hr.com/en/magazines/leadership_excellence_essentials/january_2015_leadership/six-reasons-why-leadership-training-fails-a-resear_i4mvrf4w.html

Lavoie-Tremblay, M., Fernet, C., Lavigne, G. L., & Austin, S. (2016). Transformational and abusive leadership practices: Impacts on novice nurses, quality of care and intention to leave. *Journal of Advanced Nursing, 72*(3), 582-592. https://doi.org/10.1111/jan.12860

Schuller, K. A., Kash, B. A., & Gamm, L. D. (2015). Studer Group's evidence-based leadership initiatives. *Journal of Health Organization and Management, 29*(6), 684-700. https://doi.org/10.1108/JHOM-10-2013-0211

Sherman, R. O., Bishop, M., Eggenberger, T., & Karden, R. (2007). Development of a leadership competency model. *Journal of Nursing Administration, 37*(2), 85–94. https://doi.org/10.1097/00005110-200702000-00011

Shirey, M. R. (2006). Authentic leaders creating healthy work environments for nursing practice. *American Journal of Critical Care, 15*(3), 256–276.

Swearingen, S. (2009). A journey to leadership: Designing a nursing leadership development program. *Journal of Continuing Education in Nursing, 40*(3), 107–112. https://doi.org/10.3928/00220124-20090301-02

8
Improving Patient Experience

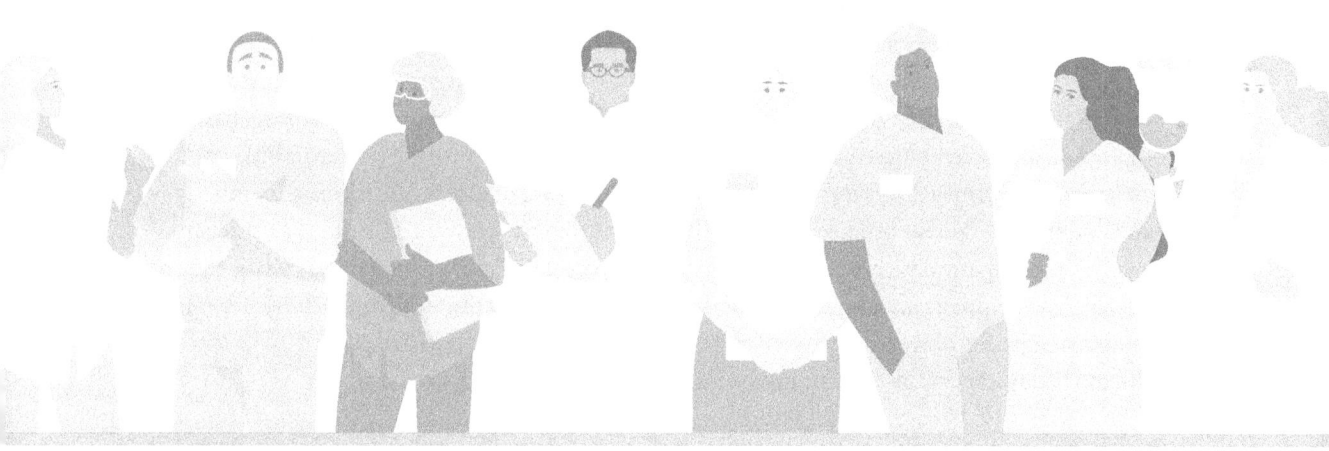

"So, we, as human beings, live in a very imprecise world. A world where our perceptions of reality are far more important than actual reality."
–Daniel Keys Moran

Many leaders in healthcare think about delivering care to patients in terms of customer service—even equating a hospital stay to a night in a hotel. When I hear this kind of language, I often feel a tightness in my chest. I just don't think of patients as customers or consumers.

For example, consider the adage "The customer is always right." That's not true of patients. When I worked in telephone triage, I received countless calls from parents who "knew" their child's ear pain was due to an ear infection and that their child needed an antibiotic. Often, however, those parents were wrong. Imagine if we allowed patients and families to assume such diagnostic roles! Our current practice of overprescribing antibiotics would reach a whole new level. Although patients and families are indeed instrumental in the diagnostic process, they do not have a license to diagnose and prescribe. (For help handling a situation like this, see Script 8.1.)

And I don't know about you, but the last time I checked into a hotel, I wasn't there seeking healthcare services, and I did not expect hotel staff to assess my pain levels, schedule medical appointments or procedures, or refer me to a specialist. All I wanted was a friendly face at the front desk, a clean room, and lots of clean, fluffy towels!

All that being said, I do see how the hotel industry—as well as the food and service industries—might shed light on service excellence initiatives in healthcare. Take Disney, for example. Disney does an outstanding job of preparing cast members to create magical experiences for their guests (Disney Institute & Kinni, 2011). Its orientation program communicates the company's culture, defines its heritage and traditions, and inspires enthusiasm among new employees, and its employee guidelines clearly and succinctly define the responsibilities of cast members. Disney also accepts corrective criticism from guests regarding cast members (and emphasizes the importance of promptly and courteously recovering from the criticism). Finally, the company clearly distinguishes between expectations of cast members when they're "onstage," when guests are present, versus "offstage" (Disney Institute & Kinni, 2011). It's no wonder many healthcare leaders who are interested in delivering positive patient experiences look to Disney's approach to customer service for guidance.

Regardless of whether you're comfortable viewing patients as customers, it's up to you to help ensure that patients at your facility have a good experience there—one where patients and families feel heard and cared for. Working toward an improved patient experience is the right thing to do—and it can pay huge dividends down the road. Healthcare organizations that do what is right for their patients thrive and flourish, even in challenging times. That's what this chapter is about.

> Like Disney cast members, healthcare workers often find themselves "onstage" and should adjust their behavior accordingly. After all, patients do not want to hear staff complaining in the cafeteria, outside patient rooms, or in hallways!

There is no "one size fits all" approach to improving patient experience. What works well in one setting or situation might not work so well in another. Make it a point to regularly evaluate and reevaluate patient experience strategies by asking patients, families, frontline staff, and other relevant stakeholders for their ideas and suggestions.

In the Driver's Seat: Perception Is Reality

For patients, perception is reality, period—and it may or may not be based on objective fact. Your perception of an interaction with a patient has meaning only if it is authenticated by the patient's perception of that interaction. For example, as a nurse, you might perceive your interaction with a patient to have been excellent. But the patient might feel you were aloof, too busy, or lacking in compassion. The patient's perception—not yours—will dictate how the patient feels about their experience at your facility. So, too, will the patient's perception of interactions with other staff. In other words, the patient might feel that *you* provided excellent care but your colleagues didn't.

A patient's perception of his experience at your organization often relates to his perception of the organization as a whole. Often, patients form this perception even before they seek treatment there. If the patient views your organization in a positive light—maybe because a friend or family member received excellent care there, or maybe because it simply has a stellar reputation—he'll likely give it the benefit of the doubt should any problems arise. If, however, he has a negative view of the organization, then every little issue, whether it's a lack of parking spaces or an encounter with a rude registrar, will seem like a big issue to him—even if he receives superior clinical care.

Complicating matters is a growing sense of consumerism among patients. I might think it's problematic to conflate patients with customers, but some patients disagree. More and more patients see healthcare as a good or service to be consumed—and they expect to leave happy from any appointment or procedure with a healthcare provider.

> The Platinum Rule plays a part in patient perception. Recall from Chapter 6 that the Platinum Rule dictates that we treat people the way *they* want to be treated, not the way *we* want to be treated (Alessandra & O'Connor, 1996).

Developing an Effective Patient Experience Strategy

In recent years, healthcare expenditures related to achieving high-quality care have increased, while public satisfaction and trust have decreased. This is largely because many of these efforts do not focus on those things that drive patient happiness. To change this—to improve patient perceptions about their experiences at your healthcare facility—you need an effective patient experience strategy.

SCRIPT 8.1
What to say when…
YOU ARE DEALING WITH ANGRY PATIENTS OR FAMILIES.

T
Time and place to talk

Choose an appropriate time and place to apologize. Find a moment when you and the person you need to apologize to can have a private conversation without distractions.

Example: Patient's Parent

> *I understand you are dissatisfied with the care you are receiving on our telephone triage line. It is our first priority to provide safe, high-quality service to everyone we care for.*

(Allow caller to vent.)

E
Explain and explore perspectives

Clearly and sincerely explain the mistake you made. Take responsibility for your actions and be honest about the impact it had on others.

Example: Angry

> *I have four children, and I know when my children have an ear infection. I don't need an appointment. I need to get an antibiotic for my child.*

> *I know it is very difficult to see your child in pain. You are correct that antibiotics are a good choice for certain diagnoses; however, an antibiotic is not the appropriate treatment if your child has an outer ear infection. (Explain swimmer's ear.) We can only determine the cause of the pain by examining the child's ear.*

L
Listen to their perspective

Allow the person to express their thoughts and feelings about the mistake. Listen attentively without interrupting, showing that you value their perspective.

Example: Still Angry

> You try dealing with a screaming child in pain! I know this cry, and it's not swimmer's ear!

> *Keeping your child comfortable is very important. (Review the treatment plan with anti-inflammatory medications, warm compress, etc.) It's important we treat your child with the most appropriate treatment plan. I highly encourage you to bring your child in for an appointment. I have an appointment available today for you.*

L
Leverage shared values and lead the conversation forward

Demonstrate your commitment to learning from the mistake and taking appropriate steps to prevent it from happening again. Share your plan for corrective action or ask for suggestions on how to rectify the situation.

Example: Still Angry

> Do you know how difficult it is for me to bring all my children out to the doctor?

> *It is very important we examine the cause of your child's pain. Can you make the appointment today?*

An effective patient strategy:

- Considers the significance of the patient's expectations with the organization's services as a whole
- Allows for the timely identification of negative perceptions
- Considers the patient experience to be of equal importance as clinical quality and patient safety
- Dedicates resources to capture, understand, and use patient experience through storytelling and numerical data
- Demonstrates an organizational commitment to understanding patient experience to improve services and co-design improvements with patients as partners
- Implements patient experience best practices

Although you may not be able to direct the perception of every patient who passes through your care, there are several important tactics you can easily implement to improve the patient experience strategy. These include taking ownership of the following:

- **Your appearance:** Looking your best creates a positive impression. Be careful not to let the stresses of the day show on your face or result in an untidy appearance. Oh—and smile!
- **Your attitude:** Choose to adopt a positive attitude before you report for work. Having a service-ready attitude tells your patients you are ready to care for them, without you even saying a word. Sometimes it's the little things we do, like acknowledging someone, that make a difference in their experience.
- **Your actions:** Practice onstage behaviors whenever you are in the sight or hearing of patients, visitors, physicians, or other guests. Examples of onstage behaviors include the following:
    - Smiling and maintaining eye contact
    - Maintaining a clean and professional appearance
    - Keeping the environment clean and uncluttered
    - Keeping the noise level down
    - Responding to questions or patient needs promptly and courteously

Onstage areas include but are not limited to the following:

- Hallways
- Nursing stations

- Procedural areas
- Patient rooms
- Cafés
- Elevators

Remember, when you're onstage, patients are the focus!

Engaging Employees and Patients

Every member of your organization plays an important role in patient experience. It's up to everyone to establish a sound relationship with every patient in the organization's care—even if it's just someone they pass in the hall. To achieve this, you need an engaged workforce.

Many healthcare organizations understand the value of an engaged workforce. In addition to heightening staff morale and benevolence, having an engaged staff can help improve patient experience. When staff feel engaged, they are more likely to go the extra mile for their patients. They are also more likely to feel confident bringing up issues that might diminish patient experience (Lindberg & Kimberlain, 2008).

Just as an engaged staff improves patient experience, so too do engaged patients. Engaged patients have improved knowledge, skills, and awareness with regard to managing their own care (Hibbard et al., 2013; Laird et al., 2015). There is also evidence that patient engagement drives better outcomes and lowers costs (Laird et al., 2015).

One way to improve patient engagement is to encourage patients and their families to play an active decision-making role. For example, suppose a new mom tells a nurse that her infant sleeps all day without waking up for feedings but won't sleep through the night. Not surprisingly, this mother is frustrated and exhausted and says she would like to start adding rice cereal to the infant's formula before bedtime so the child will sleep until morning. Rather than simply telling the new mom, "No, that could hurt your baby," the nurse listens intently and without judgment. She then clearly and kindly explains to the new mother how the extra caloric intake associated with the rice cereal could be harmful to the infant's gut and reviews other risk factors in detail. After that, the nurse and the mother review the feeding schedule to develop a better daytime routine to decrease the frequency of nighttime feeds. As a result, the new mom feels more knowledgeable and empowered to care for her baby. Had the nurse not taken the time to explain the negative effects of the rice cereal, the mom might still have fed it to her baby.

> **THE REAL WORLD**
> SCRIPTING IN PATIENT EDUCATION
>
> A study conducted by Best et al. (2017) supported that scripted preoperative pain management education for patients undergoing outpatient abdominal surgery improved patient experiences. Scripting helped standardize patient education, which in turn improved the quality of the time spent with the patient and decreased the chances of omitting important educational material.

When Mistakes Happen

Mistakes happen. When they do, it's all about the recovery. To provide consistent service recovery, Disney Institute recommends using the HEARD acronym (Disney Institute & Kinni, 2011). This acronym is also helpful for recovering from mistakes in a healthcare organization. HEARD stands for:

- **Hear:** Allow the patient to tell his whole story, without interruption. As you listen, focus not only on the patient's words, but on his body language (as well as your own). Even if you feel the patient is attacking you personally, control your emotions—not to allow the patient to be disrespectful to you, but to remind yourself to stay calm.
    - *Body language check:* Don't stand in a defensive posture with your arms crossed in front of you or your hands hiding your pelvic area (Driver & van Aalst, 2010). Also, pay attention to where your feet are positioned and how you are holding your arms. Your body language should convey warmth through a relaxed posture and an open body, sitting or standing in an appropriate proximity, and so on.

> According to the Disney Institute (Disney Institute & Kinni, 2011), when a service failure occurs, emotions rise, and customers pay more attention to how they are treated than to any recourse offered. This is why, when mistakes happen, you must acknowledge both the issue *and* the person. Be genuine, or there will be no recovery from the service failure!

- **Empathize:** By empathizing with patients, you create an emotional relationship that shows you are authentic in your willingness and ability to help. Consider scripts that validate feelings, such as the following:
    - "I understand we haven't done our best to meet your needs."
    - "I understand this is very difficult for you."

- "I see why you would be upset."
- *Body language check:* Your feet (or, if you're sitting, your knees) should point toward the patient, and your tone should be pleasant. If necessary, bring your pitch down so you don't sound condescending.

Apologize: Never underestimate the power of a sincere apology. When you apologize, be authentic, even if you personally had nothing to do with the issue at hand. You still represent the organization, so take ownership. Consider using any of these statements:

- "Please accept my apology on behalf of the organization."
- "I apologize for this inconvenience/misunderstanding/miscommunication/experience."
- "I'm so sorry we disappointed you. Our intent is to always provide you with excellent service."
- *Body language check:* Maintain eye contact and listen intently.

Resolve: Problems should be resolved instantly—or as quickly as possible. Promptness is very important to recovery. Say something like, "How can I improve this situation for you?" If the person doesn't have an answer, try one of the following statements:

- "Here is what I think we should do to improve this situation…What are your thoughts on that?"
- "Thank you for bringing this to my attention. Your comments will help us make improvements."
- *Body language check:* Again, your feet (or, if you're sitting, your knees) should point toward the patient, and your tone should be pleasant. If necessary, bring your pitch down so you don't sound condescending.

> Disney recognizes that not every service failure is due to something within its control. Even so, Disney accepts that it's the company's job to remedy the failure (Disney Institute & Kinni, 2011).

Diagnose: Setting aside guilt (yours or someone else's), consider the processes that led to the service failure.

- *Body language check:* Convey sincerity by maintaining steady eye contact and a relaxed but poised body posture and leaning or reaching toward the patient.

Script 8.2 shows how you might respond to a family member who confronts you after a mistake happens.

SCRIPT 8.2

What to say when…

YOU NEED TO APOLOGIZE TO PATIENTS OR THEIR FAMILIES.

T
Time and place to talk

Choose an appropriate time and place to have a conversation with the angry patient and their family. Find a calm and private setting where you can address their concerns without distractions.

Example: Patient or Patient's Family

> I apologize that your appointment is running two hours behind, and no one has given you an update as to when you will be seen. I would like to help in finding a solution. First, it is important that I listen to your concerns. (Allow them to vent. Use the HEARD acronym.)

> We had other doctor appointments lined up today, and now we are late because of the disorganization in appointment scheduling.

E
Explain and explore perspectives

Clearly and empathetically explain that you understand their anger and frustrations. Acknowledge their concerns and express your willingness to listen and address the issues they are experiencing.

Example: Validate and Apologize

> I would react similarly if I were in your shoes. I am very sorry, and I feel horrible that you have been here waiting for two hours.

L
Listen to their perspective

Allow the angry patient and their family to express their frustrations, concerns, and grievances. Practice active listening by giving them your full attention, maintaining eye contact, and showing empathy.

Example: Confrontational

> I want this fixed! My whole day is a mess now.

> Do you have any ideas or solutions in order to remedy this situation?

> Yes. If you can't get us in now, then we want the first appointment available tomorrow (or whatever they propose).

> Consider carefully what the family has to say, and work to provide a solution.

> *No, I don't.*

> Although I can't replace the time you lost and the inconvenience of rescheduling your other appointments, I would like to earn your trust back by offering to let you see another provider.

> Or

> I promise to continue to update you every 15 minutes about the estimated time you will be seen. We will be sure to give you the same time and attention we are giving the current cause of the delay. Safety is our top priority.

L
Leverage shared values and lead the conversation forward

Remind the angry patient and their family that your shared goal is to provide quality care and ensure their satisfaction. Emphasize that you are on the same side and committed to finding a resolution that meets their needs.

Example A: Accepting

> *Well, it's not your fault.*

> Unfortunately, emergencies happen. Being negligent of other patients' time is not acceptable. Once again, I apologize for the oversight of not keeping you well informed. In the meantime, I'd like to offer you a complimentary refreshment in the cafeteria. When you return, I will update you on the status.

Example B: Still Angry

> *I'll never come back here again!*

> Once again, I am very sorry for not keeping you well informed. In the meantime, I'd like to offer you a complimentary refreshment in the cafeteria. When you return, I will update you with the status. Unfortunately, emergencies happen. Being negligent in updating you about the appointment time is unacceptable. You can be sure you will be receiving the most comprehensive care when you are seen and given the same time and attention.

Your Road Map: Communicate, Communicate, Communicate

Realtors often say that the cardinal rule in real estate is "location, location, location." In healthcare, it's "communication, communication, communication." Healthcare is built on trusting relationships, and the cornerstone of trusting relationships is communication.

Nurses should strive to establish trusting relationships with patients and family members. Trust can take root within the first few minutes of meeting—and can wither and die in that time as well. When a patient's trust is lost, it can require a significant effort to regain it—if it can be regained at all.

One easy way to build trust is to introduce yourself by offering your name and explaining your role—and then asking the patient and family members for *their* names. All too often, nurses complete the first step but neglect the second one. Having a give-and-take relationship is cardinal to establishing trust. After all, how can you establish trust with patients and families if they don't feel like you're taking the time to learn about them? On a related note, it's not enough to ask the patient and their family to tell you their names; you must ask them to tell you their *preferred* name—and then use that name when you communicate with them. Don't wait for them to correct you! Be proactive. Get to know your patients.

Nurses can also build trust by using various communication tools and techniques that have been shown to improve patient experience (Baker, 2010; Studer, 2003; Woodard, 2009). These include AIDET, whiteboards, hourly rounding, bedside shift reporting, discharge phone calls, motivational techniques, SPIKES, measuring patient experience, and CAR.

AIDET

You may recall from Chapter 1 that AIDET, an acronym coined by the Studer Group (n.d.), is an evidence-based communication model that provides a framework for communication with patients, families, and other healthcare providers. AIDET stands for:

- **A**cknowledge
- **I**ntroduce
- **D**uration
- **E**xplanation
- **T**hank you

You can use AIDET as follows to greet patients to improve patient experience, staff satisfaction, and clinical outcomes (Studer, 2003). Notice that this approach includes crucial pieces of information designed specifically to help gain the trust of others:

- **Acknowledge:** Greet people with a smile, maintain eye contact, and demonstrate a warm, receptive attitude with everyone you meet. Be mindful, however, that direct eye contact may be disrespectful in some cultures, so you should look for cues from your patient for guidance. When in doubt, remember that a handshake or simple nod of the head is a universal sign of acknowledgment.

    Sample acknowledgment statements:

    - "Good morning, Ms. _____. We've been expecting you, and we're glad you are here."
    - "Good afternoon, Mr. _____. Welcome to Hospital ABC. We want to make your visit with us as smooth as possible. Would you please confirm that we have your most current information in this document?"

- **Introduce:** Introduce yourself by offering your name, title, and experience.

    Sample introductory statements:

    - "My name is _____, and I will be conducting your test today. I am a certified registered nurse, and I do about six of these procedures a day. Do you have any questions before we begin?"
    - "Mrs. _____, you will be seeing Dr. _____ today. He is an excellent cardiothoracic surgeon. He is renowned for his bedside manner and for thoroughly answering all questions. You are fortunate that he is your surgeon."

- **Duration:** Keep the patient informed of upcoming meals, tests, procedures, and so on. Explain how long a procedure will take, how long the patient might have to wait, or, if you are walking with someone, how long it will take to reach your destination.

    Sample duration statement:

    - "Dr. _____ has had to attend to an emergency. He wanted you to know that it may be approximately 20 minutes before he can see you. Are you able to wait, or would you like me to schedule an appointment for tomorrow?"

- **Explanation:** Explain to patients what they can expect before, during, and after a test or procedure.

    Sample explanation statement:

    - "I want to explain a little more about your procedure. We are performing it because _____. What will happen is _____. You may experience side effects like _____. Do you have any questions?"

- **Thank you:** Sincerely thank patients, families, and visitors for choosing your hospital and for trusting you to provide care. Be polite and use direct eye contact.

    Sample thank-you statements:

    - "Thank you for choosing Hospital ABC and trusting us to meet your healthcare needs. It has been a privilege to care for you."
    - "Thank you for calling us. Is there anything else I can do for you? I have the time."

> If you are using an interpreter, body language can also help put the patient at ease and develop trust in the staff.

Using AIDET for Pain Management

Some acronyms can be used in multiple ways. For example, in addition to using AIDET to greet patients, you could use it for the purposes of pain management (Studer, 2003) as follows:

- **Acknowledge:** Acknowledge when you see a patient in pain—for example, "Mr. Jones, you look very uncomfortable."
- **Introduce:** Introduce the topic of the importance of pain management and express your concern as to whether the patient's pain level is tolerable.
- **Duration:** Indicate the duration of the proposed pain-management medication's effectiveness and how the dosing is scheduled.
- **Explanation:** Explain to the patient why you're doing what you're doing—for example, why you are administering certain medications, treatments, or care plans.
- **Thank you:** Thank the patient for trusting in you.

Whiteboards

The placement of whiteboards in patient rooms is an increasingly common tactic to improve communication (Sehgal et al., 2010). These boards allow any number of care providers to communicate a wide range of information. Here are some tips for using whiteboards:

- Position the whiteboard in clear view of the patient from his hospital bed.
- Attach an erasable pen to the whiteboard and keep a supply of fresh pens at the nursing station to replace missing or fading ones.

- Create a whiteboard template to ensure the whiteboard conveys both important and accurate information, such as the name of the patient's current caregiver and the patient's goals for the day. A blank whiteboard reduces standardization in practice and fails to remind providers to write and review content on the whiteboard.

- Ensure the care team regularly updates the whiteboard. Leaving the whiteboard empty or outdated sends a message to the patient that the staff is not paying attention to detail, they're too busy, or they simply don't think updating the board is important. Remember: Members of the clinical team may pass by the whiteboard many times per shift, but the patient is basically staring at it all day.

> Pay attention to details like these. Patients and families do!

I presume some of these tips are already hardwired into your daily practice, but you'd be surprised how often this is not the case. While speaking to nurse audiences about patient experience, I often ask, "How many of you write down goals on the whiteboard?" Inevitably, almost every nurse in the audience raises their hand. But when I ask, "How many nurses write down the *patient's* goals?" I don't see so many raised hands.

The goals of a caregiver are often quite different from those of a patient or family member. For example, the goal of an NICU nurse might be to advance tube feeding by 2 ccs every other hour. However, I highly doubt the patient's mother has the same goal. More likely, her goal is to hold her baby. If that's not possible—for example, if the baby is in the incubator due to temperature intolerance—the nurse could compromise and tell the mother that she can do the next diaper change with the nurse's help, or, if the mother is nervous about changing the diaper because of the number of cords attached to the baby, she can hold the baby's foot or hand while the nurse changes the baby's diaper.

> Ask the patient (or family) what their goals are, make a list, and keep it on the patient's whiteboard. Then, review and check off the goals on a continual basis, such as when you do hourly rounds. Note that this is a wonderful way to keep other caregivers in the loop, too.

Hourly Rounds

Nurse continuity is an important aspect of patient experience. So, too, is consistent and purposeful nurse-patient rounding (Blakley et al., 2011). Simply put, nurses who consistently and purposefully conduct rounds proactively care for patients. In contrast, nurses who don't round consistently and purposefully find that nurse call buttons are used more frequently, at various times, and for various reasons (Harrington et al., 2013).

Some hospitals have adopted the Four Ps approach for purposeful rounding (Woodard, 2009). Nurses who take this approach ask the following four questions every hour the patient is awake:

- **Pain:** "How is your pain?"
- **Position:** "Are you comfortable?"
- **Potty:** "Do you need to use the bathroom?"
- **Presence:** "Is there anything I can get you, such as the call light, phone, trash can, water, or over-bed table?"

> Coaching nurses to make time to authentically listen to patients is mutually beneficial. Patients who feel heard are less likely to monopolize what time we can devote to them.

Patients should feel that their feedback is both welcomed and considered.

THE REAL WORLD
THE POSITIVE IMPACT OF HOURLY PATIENT ROUNDING

Sacred Heart, a 476-bed acute care facility located in Pensacola, Florida, USA, implemented hourly rounding in 10 of its nursing units. Five months into implementation, here were the results (Studer Group, 2007):

- Call light use decreased by 40%–50%.
- Patient falls decreased by 33%.
- Hospital-acquired pressure ulcer cases decreased by 56%.
- Overall patient satisfaction increased by 71%.

Bedside Shift-Change Reporting

Bedside shift-change reporting is when nurses conduct shift-change reports at the patient's bedside. This practice enables patients to be more engaged and instrumental in their care by ensuring accurate information is shared among all healthcare members. Patients can also elect a family member or close friend to participate.

Bedside reporting need not be limited to shift changes. It's also useful for introducing a replacement RN or care extender (medical assistant, licensed practical nurse, and so on) when primary nurses need to leave the floor for lunch breaks or to take other patients to various departments.

Bedside shift reports have many benefits, including improved:

- Communication
- Participation in setting care goals
- Opportunity for patients to ask questions and share experiences
- Safe patient handoff and information-gathering
- Assessment of patient's surgical wounds, pressure ulcers, and so on
- Patient and caregiver trust (by confirming nurses are conveying information properly)
- Team accountability (by encouraging a successful transition to practice environment for nurses)

Here are some tips for effective bedside shift-change reports:

- Start the report by using AIDET to introduce the staff to the patient and family members.
- Ask the patient about her preferences—for example, whether family members and/or visitors should leave the room during the report.
- Ask for the patient's input and maintain a triangular stance to avoid excluding the patient during the report.
- Increase patient confidence by letting her know that a great nurse or provider will be taking care of her.
- Discuss clinical care issues and provide clinical updates—for example, patient information, laboratory results, wound care, medications, and so on.
- Discuss care goals for the next shift.
- Answer questions from the patient or family members (or write the questions down to be addressed at a later time) and address unresolved issues.
- Update information on the whiteboard, such as the incoming nurse's and assistant's names, treatment goals, patient goals, anticipated discharge date, and so on.

THE REAL WORLD
EMBRACING CRITICAL CONVERSATIONS TO IMPROVE PATIENT CARE

At PeaceHealth St. Joseph Medical Center, administrators launched a Safe to Speak Up campaign to promote communication and transparency in the organization. They wanted to create a safe environment where staff felt empowered to engage in honest and transparent communication. This campaign embraces critical conversations among caregivers, which is the cornerstone for superior patient-centered care.

Discharge Phone Calls

Because many patients are anxious to get home after a hospital stay, they don't always take the time to fully understand the instructions given during discharge. Discharge phone calls are a terrific way to reinforce these instructions, further educate patients about their treatment plan, and generally follow up. Discharge phone calls also give patients an opportunity to double-check instructions, which may help minimize calls to providers or even emergency department visits in the future. Finally, discharge calls can aid in service recovery. After all, the average patient can't judge the total quality of their healthcare experience until after they are discharged.

Discharge phone calls are intended to maximize the patient experience—not necessarily provide medical advice. Still, during these calls, nurses should ask the patient follow-up questions such as the following:

- Does the patient understand all the discharge instructions provided?
- Has the patient filled prescriptions?
- Does the patient have questions about medications?
- Does the patient have any pain related to the diagnosis?
- Has the patient made follow-up appointments?
- How does the patient feel about the care they received, and do they think anything could have been done differently?

The nurse should document all information obtained from the discharge call and refer patients who have clinical questions or are experiencing a medical problem to their physician or care provider as appropriate. Even if the patient doesn't have clinical questions and is not experiencing a medical problem, the nurse should loop back to the physician team to let them know the results of the call. Finally, the nurse should forward information about the patient's perception of care to management as a learning opportunity and so that an action plan for service recovery can be implemented.

Motivating Patients to Care for Themselves

Taking a motivational approach can be very effective for improving patient outcomes. For example, suppose your patient is not taking his medications properly. Taking a motivational approach can empower him to change his ineffective habits by exploring and resolving any ambivalence he may have. When you take this approach, patients change their behavior because they want to, not because you or the doctor told them to. Simply put, when patients have a better understanding of "what's in it for them," they are more apt to comply with their care regimen (Miller & Rollnick, 2013).

Positive reinforcement is also key to patient care. Consider the meaningful-use questions required by the Centers for Medicare & Medicaid Services (CMS), which call for healthcare providers to ask whether patients smoke. When a patient says no, many healthcare providers simply check that box on the electronic health record and continue to the next question. Instead, they should reinforce the patient's behavior by observing that the patient is making a healthy choice by refraining from smoking.

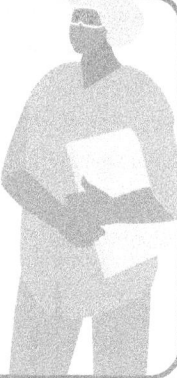

Time to Reflect

How many times a day do you provide positive reinforcement to your patients and/or staff? Is there room to improve?

You can use the TELL acronym to motivate patients:

- **T – Time and place to talk:** Choose an appropriate time and place for the conversation where both parties can have privacy.
- **E – Explain and explore perspectives:** Explain the positive aspects for the change, such as how the things the patient values in life will be improved.
- **L – Listen to their perspective:** Allow the patient to share how they see the situation. Take time to pause and listen.
- **L – Leverage shared values and lead the conversation forward:** Use positive reinforcement and highlight how this behavioral change will positively influence what's most important to them.

Using SPIKES to Deliver Bad News

According to Buckman (2005) and Kaplan (2010), some healthcare professionals use the SPIKES acronym when delivering bad news to cancer patients. This acronym helps clinicians meet the main objectives when delivering the information. These include the following:

- Gathering information from the patient
- Transmitting medical information
- Providing support to the patient
- Obtaining the patient's cooperation and collaboration in the treatment plan

SPIKES stands for the following:

- **Setting:** Be sure the patient has with her any family she wants present and that you are meeting at a time when interruptions will be limited.
- **Perception:** This relates to how doctors determine what patients already know and how much they *want* to know.
- **Invitation:** Not everyone wants to know everything. Let the patient invite you to provide more information.
- **Knowledge:** Use layman's terms—words that the patient and family members can understand. For example, instead of using the word "metastasize," use the word "spread."
- **Empathetic response:** Be empathetic. Pay attention to the patient's emotional reactions.
- **Strategy:** Outline the next several steps of the treatment plan.

Time to Reflect

Ms. Anderson is a previously healthy 50-year-old accountant who initially presented with a seizure. A CT scan showed an enhancing mass, and the patient was referred to a neurosurgeon for a biopsy. Consider the following:

- How would you convey empathy?
- How can you help the patient and her family feel integrated in the patient's care?

Delivering bad news is never easy. However, by preparing for these conversations, you can make them less burdensome and more effective. Keep these tips in mind:

- Avoid reassuring phrases like "Don't worry" or "It'll all be OK." Phrases like these may make it more difficult for patients to accept their diagnosis, treatment plan, and transition of care.
- Breathe and observe your body language. Lower your shoulders and uncross your arms. If you notice you're experiencing anxious thoughts, breathe more deeply.
- Listen with respect and patience. Strive to understand and appreciate what the patient is going through and to find something to connect with for further discussion. Instead of trying to escape the patient's emotional experience, imagine the emotions are an ocean wave that will flow over you safely. The wave does not have to knock you over like a tsunami.

- Keep your tone of voice calm and avoid persuading, convincing, or arguing with patients and families.
- Be willing to acknowledge further steps such as stating, "This is a first step."

Measuring Patient Experience

The Hospital Consumer Assessment of Healthcare Providers and Systems (HCAHPS) survey is the first national, standardized, publicly reported survey instrument of patient perspectives of hospital care. HCAHPS measures how well healthcare providers as a team met patient expectations, how satisfied patients were with their visit or stay, and how well the outcomes the patient expected were delivered both clinically and experientially. It then compares hospital performance on a local, regional, and national level (HCAHPS, 2012).

The HCAHPS survey asks discharged patients about their recent hospital experience. It contains questions about various aspects of the patient's hospital experience, including communication with nurses and doctors, responsiveness of hospital staff, cleanliness and quietness of the hospital environment, pain management, communication about medicines, discharge information, overall rating of the hospital, and likelihood that the patient would recommend the hospital to others (CMS, 2013). Hospitals can use the HCAHPS survey on its own or can include additional questions.

> Consider forming a committee whose job is to help the healthcare facility improve HCAHPS scores.

Administering the HCAHPS Survey

The HCAHPS survey is administered via random sampling of adult patients with varying medical conditions between 48 hours and six weeks after discharge. Hospitals may use an approved survey vendor or collect their own HCAHPS data (with the approval of CMS). Surveys must be conducted throughout each month of the year.

Survey vendors and hospitals execute the HCAHPS survey using four different methods:

- Mail
- Telephone
- Mail with telephone follow-up
- Interactive voice response

For more information about the HCAHPS survey, visit http://www.hcahpsonline.org.

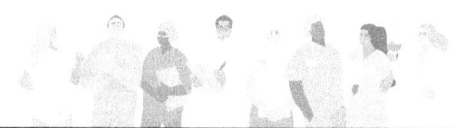

The goal for care facilities is to earn "top box" ratings, or the highest ratings possible, for each item on the HCAHPS survey (CMS, 2013). This is no small feat, in part because patients rate their experience based on their perception—which, as discussed, may differ greatly from the perception of various caregivers.

In 2013, HCAHPS scores became one of 13 measures used by CMS to calculate $850 million in payments from its new value-based purchasing (VBP) program. Thirty percent of the VBP score is based on HCAHPS, with the rest based on clinical measures. To protect their CMS reimbursements, many hospitals and health systems have initiated strategies to improve not only their scores on each of the core questions but also overall patient experience (CMS, 2013). This is especially critical as healthcare systems face many financial uncertainties (Hall, 2008). These strategies include comprehensive leadership training and employee experience initiatives.

All nurses should become familiar with HCAHPS questions. This can help them fine-tune their care to address issues covered by the survey. Following are examples of HCAHPS questions, as well as scripts you can use to provide excellent patient care and customer service (while maintaining a budget) to improve the likelihood that patients will give your organization the best possible rating (Reynolds, 2013).

- **HCAHPS question:** "How often did nurses listen carefully to you?"

    Scripting:

    - "It sounds like you're worried/concerned about _____. Can you tell me more about how you're feeling?"
    - "I know you have received a lot of information today. Can you tell me what you understood?"
    - "I know you've discussed _____ with your physician. Can you tell me about any worries or concerns you have?"

- **HCAHPS question:** "How often did hospital staff describe possible side effects in a way you could understand?"

    Scripting:

    - "Your doctor prescribed [medication] to [regulate/manage/decrease/increase] your [symptom]. Before you take this medication, I want to be sure you are clear as to why it is important for you. If a loved one were to ask you why you are taking this medication, how would you answer them?"

> Like AIDET, HCAHPS scripts can also be modified for multiple uses—for example, by front-desk staff, housekeeping, admissions, and all interdisciplinary departments. HCAHPS scripting need not apply just to the nursing department; after all, this survey is meant to assess the performance of all staff who meet and greet patients.

- **HCAHPS question:** "Before giving you any new medicine, how often did hospital staff describe possible side effects in a way you could understand?"

Scripting:

- "We started you on [medication]. Can you tell me at what time you will take it each day and what it's for?"
- "What side effects would tell you to call your doctor?"

Half of the core questions in the HCAHPS survey pertain to communication—how patients perceived interactions with nurses, doctors, and other hospital staff. This means it's particularly vital for nurses to effectively communicate with patients. Small acts of kindness, like taking time to build trusting relationships, reap big rewards.

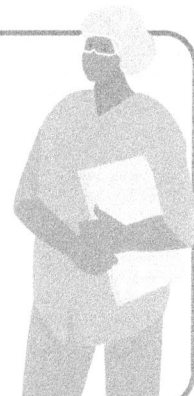

Time to Reflect

HCAHPS scores should be transparent. To assess how transparent your hospital's HCAHPS scores are, use the ARE acronym:

- **A**ccurate
- **R**eadily available
- **E**asy to access

Using the CAR Approach to Communicate With Patients

When nurses communicate with patients, incorporating the CAR approach ensures that key talking points are addressed and that body language and emotions are considered. This approach also helps garner more productive and comprehensive discussions.

- **Consideration:** Consider your attitude, tone, and pitch. Are your emotions in check? Are you hastily caring for the patient or feverishly asking questions because something else is on your mind? Also consider the Five Rights of Communication Safety. When the patient speaks, actively listen to their concerns and reflectively respond to or address them accordingly, without multitasking. Sitting with the patient rather than standing increases the patient's perception of the duration of your conversation.

- **Action or call to action:** Determine your action or call to action. This involves being an active listener and following through on answers received. Follow the QWQ formula (see Chapter 2) to allow the patient adequate time to formulate an answer. Use the whiteboard to document the patient's targeted pain score for nursing staff. Listen for medication effectiveness, interactions, and interventions that might be needed. Combining scripting and teach-back enables nurses to achieve higher levels of therapeutic interaction and patient experience.

- **Return on investment (ROI):** This is the amount of time you invest in the patient. Quality of time rather than quantity of time is key. Determine whether there is anything else you could ask or do for the patient. Make the ROI worth the investment by earning the trust of your patients and their families.

The Drive Home

Let's drive home the key points in this chapter:

- Healthcare organizations that do what is right for their patients thrive and flourish, even in challenging times.

- Patient perceptions stem from all the experiences they had before, during, and after hospitalization.

- Individual employees directly influence patient perceptions. Therefore, each encounter is critical. It is not enough to satisfy patients some of the time. Healthcare providers must consistently satisfy patients with every interaction.

- Communication tools and techniques have been shown to improve patient experience. These include using AIDET to greet patients, whiteboards to communicate important information to the patient and the staff, hourly rounding, bedside shift changes, discharge phone calls, motivation and positive reinforcement, SPIKES to deliver bad news, measuring patient experience, and incorporating the CAR approach.

- HCAHPS is a standardized survey that provides information about the patient's experience and quality of care. This information is publicly reported.

References

Alessandra, T., & O'Connor, M. J. (1996). *The Platinum Rule: Discover the four basic business personalities—and how they can lead you to success.* Grand Central Publishing.

Baker, S. J. (2010). Bedside shift report improves patient safety and nurse accountability. *Journal of Emergency Nursing, 36*(4), 355–358. https://doi.org/10.1016/j.jen.2010.03.009

Best, J. T., Musgrave, B., Pratt, K., Hill, R., Evans, C., & Corbitt, D. (2017). The impact of scripted pain education on patient satisfaction in outpatient abdominal surgery patients. *Journal of PeriAnesthesia Nursing, 33*(4), P452–460. https://doi.org/10.1016/j.jopan.2016.02.014

Blakley, D., Kroth, M., & Gregson, J. (2011). The impact of nurse rounding on patient satisfaction in a medical-surgical hospital unit. *Medsurg Nursing, 20*(6), 327–332.

Buckman, R. A. (2005). Breaking bad news: The S-P-I-K-E-S strategy. *Community Oncology, 2*(2), 138–142. https://doi.org/10.1016/S1548-5315(11)70867-1

Centers for Medicare & Medicaid Services. (2013). *HCAHPS.* http://www.hcahpsonline.org

Disney Institute, & Kinni, T. (2011). *Be our guest: Perfecting the art of customer service.* Disney Editions.

Driver, J., & van Aalst, M. (2010). *You say more than you think: A 7-day plan for using the new body language to get what you want.* Crown Publishers.

Hall, M. F. (2008). Looking to improve financial results? Start by listening to patients. *Healthcare Financial Management, 62*(10), 76–80.

Harrington, A., Bradley, S., Jeffers, L., Linedale, E., Kelman, S., & Killington, G. (2013). The implementation of intentional rounding using participatory action research. *International Journal of Nursing Practice, 19*(5), 523–529. https://doi.org/10.1111/ijn.12101

Hibbard, J. H., Greene, J., & Overton, V. (2013). Patients with lower activation associated with higher costs; delivery systems should know their patients' 'scores'. *Health Affairs, 2*(32), 216–222. https://doi.org/10.1377/hlthaff.2012.1064

Hospital Consumer Assessment of Healthcare Providers and Systems. (2012). *Autumn 2012 HCAHPS executive insight letter.* http://www.hcahpsonline.org/globalassets/hcahps/executive-insight/2012-autumn-hei-letter.pdf

Kaplan, M. (2010). SPIKES: A framework for breaking bad news to patients with cancer. *Clinical Journal of Oncology Nursing, 14*(4), 514–516. https://doi.org/10.1188/10.CJON.514-516

Laird, E. A., McCance, T., McCormack, B., & Gribben, B. (2015). Patients' experiences of in-hospital care when nursing staff were engaged in a practice development programme to promote person-centredness: A narrative analysis study. *International Journal of Nursing Studies, 52*(9), 1454–1462. https://doi.org/10.1016/j.ijnurstu.2015.05.002

Lindberg, L., & Kimberlain, J. (2008). Quality update: Engage employees to improve staff and patient satisfaction. *Hospitals & Health Networks, 82*(1), 28–29.

Miller, W. R., & Rollnick, S. (2013.) *Motivational interviewing: Helping people change.* The Guilford Press.

Reynolds, A. (2013, June). *Setting yourself and your patients up for success: Utilizing scripting in the OB setting.* Poster presentation at the 2013 AWHONN Convention, Nashville, TN.

Sehgal, N. L., Green, A., Vidyarhi, A. R., Blegen, M. A., & Wachter, R. M. (2010). Patient whiteboards as a communication tool in the hospital setting: A survey of practices and recommendations. *Journal of Hospital Medicine, 5*(4), 234–239. https://doi.org/10.1002/jhm.638

Studer Group. (n.d.). *AIDET patient communication.* http://www.studergroup.com/aidet

Studer Group. (2007). *Hourly rounding supplement: Best practice: Sacred Heart Hospital, Pensacola, Florida.* Author.

Studer, Q. (2003). *Hardwiring excellence: Purpose, worthwhile work, making a difference.* Fire Starter Publishing.

Woodard, J. L. (2009). Effects of rounding on patient satisfaction and patient safety on a medical-surgical unit. *Clinical Nurse Specialist, 23*(4), 200–206. https://doi.org/10.1097/NUR.0b013e3181a8ca8a

9

Fostering a Healthy Workplace Environment

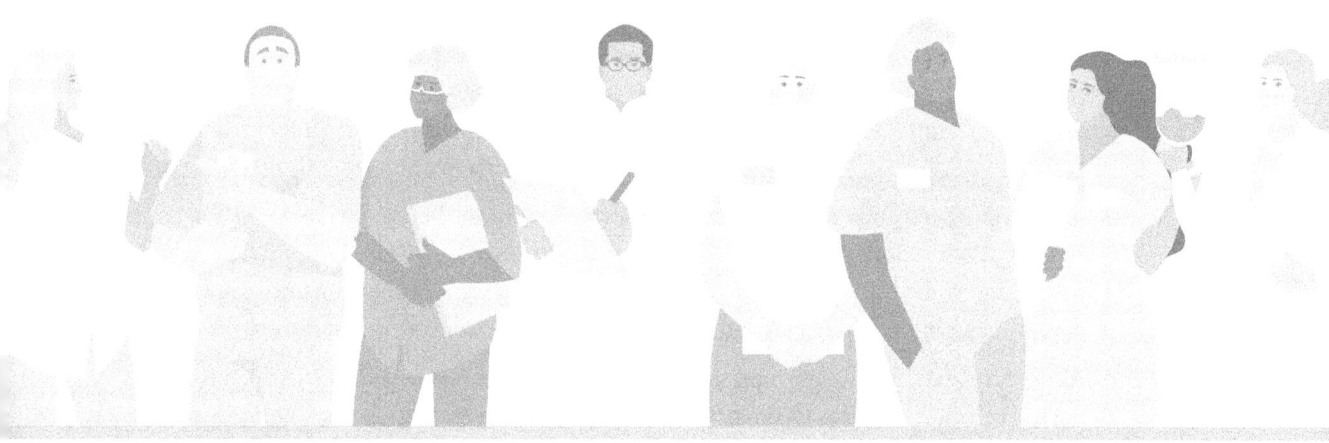

"Going to work for a large company is like getting on a train. Are you going 60 miles an hour, or is the train going 60 miles an hour and you're just sitting still?"
–J. Paul Getty

The definition of a healthy workplace has evolved considerably over the years. It originally focused almost exclusively on the physical work environment. Now, however, the definition has expanded to include interpersonal and psychosocial factors as well as environmental issues—all of which can have a profound effect on employee health and workplace satisfaction (Blake, 2016; Cummings et al., 2010).

These days, a healthy workplace environment (HWE) provides staff a feeling of inclusion, safety, and motivation. The staff cares about the organization because they feel it has their best interests at heart. An HWE in a healthcare setting encourages better teamwork, increased productivity, improved patient experience scores and safety outcomes, and decreased sick leave and employee attrition rates. And, of course, it's much easier to have critical conversations in nursing when you operate in an HWE!

The American Association of Critical-Care Nurses (AACN) has developed six standards for establishing and sustaining an HWE (AACN, 2016):

- **Skilled communication:** According to The Joint Commission, poor communication is a leading contributor to sentinel events. Healthcare organizations are encouraged to identify and address barriers to effective communication among healthcare teams.

- **True collaboration:** True collaboration means walking the talk—in other words, engaging in actions that support words. True collaboration is a process, not an isolated event. True collaboration also means giving credit where credit is due—and not taking it when it's not deserved. (Script 9.1 outlines how to handle when someone claims credit for your idea.)

- **Effective decision-making:** Nurses who do not have control over their scope of practice feel marginalized and demoralized. It's critical to empower them to make decisions. Nurses must also be educated in the skills of communication, goal-setting, negotiation, conflict management and resolution, and performance improvement. Education and professional development in these skills are key to successfully implementing this standard.

- **Appropriate staffing:** Inappropriate staffing compromises patient safety—which is *always* the top priority—and is a leading cause of dissatisfaction among nurses. With the increasing complexity of patient illnesses, appropriate staffing involves more than just a fixed nurse-to-patient ratio. (Note that ensuring that the standards of true collaboration and effective decision-making are met can help bridge staffing gaps.)

- **Meaningful recognition:** For nurses to feel valued by the organization, they must be recognized by the organization for their contributions and performance. They must also take an active role in recognizing their peers and colleagues in kind.

- **Authentic leadership:** Authentic leaders adopt flexible styles that fit the situation and capabilities of their teammates. These leaders are also genuine—remaining sensitive to the needs of others while adjusting their behavior according to the context.

These six standards reflect evidence-based and relationship-centered principles of professional performance. Only when healthcare professionals, organizations, and professional associations adopt these standards can the journey to an HWE begin (AACN, 2016).

In the Driver's Seat: Embracing Change

According to Blake (2016), there are several barriers to implementing and sustaining an HWE. These include poor collaboration, inadequate staffing, and a lack of accountability and meaningful recognition. In essence, creating an HWE requires changing long-standing cultures, traditions, and hierarchies—which, like all types of change, is very difficult.

Change Management Versus Change Leadership

As we discuss change, it is important to clarify the distinction between change management and change leadership. *Change management* refers to a set of basic tools or configurations intended to keep a change initiative under the control of someone or something. The goal of change management is often to decrease interruptions and to soften the effects of the change. In contrast, *change leadership* focuses on the strategic process that facilitates a comprehensive transformation. Change leadership is key to improving patient experience and employee satisfaction, and thus sustaining an HWE.

Many healthcare organizations seek to implement these and other changes. And yet, according to LaClair and Rao (2002), about 70% of all change initiatives in all organizations end in failure. Here are some key reasons why:

> **"Hurry up and wait":** Have you ever rushed to be on time for a doctor's appointment, only to find out when you get there that the doctor is running 20 minutes behind? This type of "hurry up and wait" experience can be beyond frustrating! Healthcare leaders often experience a similar "hurry up and wait" scenario. To keep up with the competition in the marketplace, they feel pressure to implement improvements across the organization to get that competitive edge. So, they "hurry up" to push out change initiatives without conducting the appropriate research or offering sufficient support for the staff charged with implementing the change. The result is that they often wind up frustrated because they are looking for a short-term solution for a long-term problem. Here's an example: Suppose a hospital's marketing team decides to advertise emergency department (ED) patient wait times on the organization's website in an effort to increase ED traffic. In their rush to implement this new feature, however, the marketing team failed to thoroughly investigate whether ED wait times tended to be high or low. Nor did they call for an increase in ED staff to handle the desired higher patient throughput. As a result, when potential patients

used the new website feature to check the wait time, they discovered the wait time was quite high and went elsewhere. The lesson: Had the marketing team been in less of a hurry to implement this change, the initiative would likely have been more successful.

- **Knowledge deficit (or not):** Leaders often think the foundational issue underlying some larger problem is a lack of knowledge, so they implement change initiatives to improve knowledge levels. Often, however, the *real* issue is whether what people do reflects what they know. The truth is, there is often a gap between what people know and what they do. For example, suppose a nonclinical leader in charge of operations informs a nurse manager that the most recent data indicate that the number of occupied beds in his unit is down; therefore, he needs to decrease staffing. The nurse manager realizes that although the number of occupied beds is indeed down, patient acuity is up. However, for fear of getting into trouble by arguing this point, he begins canceling staff, resulting in unsafe patient ratios. In other words, despite knowing it's a bad idea to decrease staffing, the nurse manager does it anyway. Eliminating this gap between what we know and what we do is critical to fostering an HWE.

- **Lack of practice:** Too many managers confuse knowledge with skill. They don't realize that it's not enough to *know* something; you must practice that thing to become skilled at it. This often happens when organizations institute a change initiative that involves nurses attending training classes. Their manager expects exceptional results the minute they walk out of the class, but that's not realistic. As with sports, music, or anything else, you must practice to improve.

- **Negative culture:** A negative culture can stymie attempts at change. Often this is because the rank and file don't feel comfortable voicing their opinions about the proposed change—negative or positive—to leadership. A nurse manager once told me she was warned early in her new job never to criticize her chief nursing officer's (CNO's) ideas—even if the CNO gave permission to do so—or risk career suicide. In that kind of culture, just about any change initiative will be doomed to failure.

- **Lack of commitment:** Everyone knows they're supposed to eat well and exercise. Yet all too often we order fries and skip the gym—and then complain about gaining weight. The same thing happens in organizations. Healthcare organizations state that their number-one goal is to improve the patient experience (Pund & Sklar, 2012). But do they do everything they can to make this happen—such as improving the staffing matrix, providing leadership training, recognizing staff, providing coaching and mentoring for succession planning, and so on? No. Take leadership training, for example. Research shows that effectively integrating leadership training into nursing has a positive impact on nurse retention rates and patient outcomes (Cowden et al., 2011), and yet there is strong evidence that leadership training needs further development (Kelly et al., 2014).

> **Time to Reflect**
>
> To improve your odds for a successful change initiative, consider the following:
>
> - Are change goals specific, measurable, attainable, relevant, and time-bound (SMART; Meyer, 2003)?
> - Is the change initiative supported by the CNO, chief executive officer (CEO), or chief operating officer (COO)?
> - Do senior leaders walk the talk?
> - Do middle managers and supervisors understand why change is needed?
> - Is the organization invested in the change initiative for the long haul?

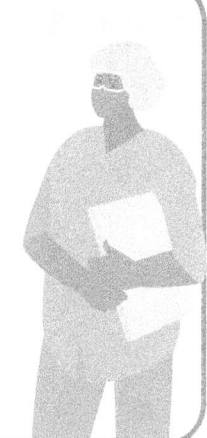

Your Road Map: Building an HWE Starts With You

Members of both formal and informal leadership share a responsibility to create a positive work environment where staff enjoy coming to work and patients feel safe and valued. To achieve this, Geedey (2006) suggests the following:

- Encourage humor.
- Clearly define unit values and expectations.
- Maintain an organized and uncluttered workspace.
- Recognize and promote volunteerism.

Yes, some major change initiatives must start at the top—meaning there is commitment from the CNO, COO, and/or CEO. But changes like these can be made at any level. Indeed, if you follow these tips, you may be shocked by what you can achieve—regardless of your title. Beyond that, building an HWE involves establishing committees to drive desired changes, obtaining buy-in by motivating others, transformational leadership, and a culture of ownership.

SCRIPT 9.1

What to say when…

YOU NEED TO TELL YOUR SUPERVISOR SOMEONE ELSE TOOK CREDIT FOR YOUR WORK.

T
Time and place to talk

Choose an appropriate time and place to have a conversation with your supervisor. Find a quiet and private setting where you can discuss the issue without interruptions.

> *Tony, I would like to speak with you about something a little uncomfortable. I am very supportive of teamwork, so I am concerned when my colleagues don't work well as a team. When is a good time to meet?*

E
Explain and explore perspectives

Clearly and calmly explain the situation to your supervisor, providing specific details about how someone else took credit for your work. Be objective and stick to the facts.

Example A: Supportive

> *Sure, let's meet now.*

> *Specifically, I am concerned about Connie's comments in today's meeting when she said her abstract was accepted for podium presentation at this year's regional Nursing Excellence Conference.*

Example B: Downplaying Concerns

> *You know, I don't like tattletales and other juvenile behavior. We are a team, after all.*

> *I agree we are a team. As a member of the team, I don't like it when hard work is not recognized or when it is undermined. Team members shouldn't disrespect their teammates.*

L
Listen to Their Perspective

Allow your supervisor to share their thoughts and gather their perspective on the situation. Listen actively and be open to their feedback or insights.

Example A: Supportive

> *Right, what is the problem?*

I came up with the abstract's idea a few months ago. I told Connie all about my idea in hopes of working with her on this, but she said my idea wasn't strong enough to submit for the conference. I have a few emails here to show you I originated the idea. I'm sad that she took my idea and didn't include me in her plans. I feel betrayed. And I thought it was important that you knew the truth.

Example B: Unsupportive

I'm sure Connie didn't mean to disrespect you. You also have to consider she could have built upon your original idea, making it completely different.

I told Connie all about my idea in hopes to work with her on this, but she said my idea wasn't strong enough to submit for the conference. I have a few emails here to show you I originated the idea—the idea she submitted. I'm sad that she took my idea and didn't include me in her plans. I feel betrayed. And I thought it was important you know how much work I put into this. I just wanted you to be aware of her behavior and my contributions.

L
Leverage shared values and lead the conversation forward

Remind your supervisor of the shared goals and values within the workplace, such as fairness, recognition, and teamwork. Emphasize the importance of accurate recognition and the impact it has on the overall work environment.

Example A: Receptive

I'll speak with Connie if you'd like. I'm sorry you were slighted.

Thank you for listening and for your support. I would like to have a meeting with you and Connie to discuss this.

Example B: Unreceptive

I think you're taking this out of context. It's not that big of a deal.

I'm concerned other nurses may not submit ideas in the future because the unit is working in silos, and there's an unhealthy atmosphere of competitiveness.

Establishing Key Committees

To build an HWE, your organization will need to field several steering committees. These committees could focus on the following. (I'll talk more about each of these types of committees and share some ideas for you to consider in a moment.)

- Rewards and recognition
- Hiring right
- Transformational rounding
- Discharge follow-up
- Welcoming new recruits
- Leadership training and education
- Physician and staff engagement
- "Bright ideas"

Before I start any project, I remember the five Ps of performance: Proper planning prevents poor performance. The same goes for forming committees. To ensure these committees perform well, you must plan ahead.

One aspect of planning ahead is considering the composition of these committees. Each committee should be composed of a cross-section of staff at every level—including members of senior leadership. This will demonstrate management's commitment to the cause and prevent the over-emphasis of "employee satisfiers," such as free coffee, cafeteria vouchers, and extra vacation time (Brunges & Foley-Brinza, 2014).

It's also critical that you choose the right champions to lead each committee. To ensure staff engagement, activate your "early adopters" in this role—the ones who are passionate about the committee's mission. They will influence and motivate others to get involved.

As for the logistics—number of members, how members are selected, meeting times, tools used, and so on—that all depends on the organization's culture and policies, so I won't get into that here.

> It's a good policy to encourage all staff to sign up for at least one committee. To ensure maximum participation and engagement, I suggest you take a "what's in it for me" approach. That is, when calling on staff to volunteer, frame it in such a way to reflect how doing so will help *them*. That is, don't just send out an email or hold a town hall meeting and ask your staff to join a committee. Instead, spell out specific benefits that committee members will enjoy.

Forming, Storming, Norming, and Performing

Psychologist Bruce Tuckman (1965) observed that committees, teams, and other types of groups go through four main phases as they develop: forming, storming, norming, and performing.

During the first stage, forming, group members are positive and polite. Some members are anxious because they don't know each other or haven't worked out what their individual contribution to the committee will be. Discussions during this stage often center around group processes, which may frustrate those group members who are more action-oriented (Smith, 2005). According to Tuckman, this stage is usually brief—often lasting only until the introductory meeting is complete.

Soon, emotions start percolating. Let the storming phase begin! During this phase, the group defines its action plan. It also assigns various roles to individuals within the group—including leadership roles. This phase may involve some conflict as members debate their own roles and the direction of the committee. Many groups fail during this phase. It's critical that your group stay motivated and focused.

Next, the committee moves into a norming stage. During this stage, group members become better acquainted. They feel more comfortable asking for help from each other and providing constructive criticism when appropriate. They also socialize more. This builds cohesion and increases the likelihood of success.

Finally, the group enters the performing phase. This is when the group's hard work results in the creation of their shared vision. By this phase, the group's culture has been established. Therefore, even if group members leave or new members join, the group's culture will remain intact (Smith, 2005).

Remember: Forming, storming, and norming need to happen before the group can start performing!

Rewards and Recognition

Recognizing good work is a great way to foster an HWE. Unfortunately, this practice is often overlooked. Indeed, according to a 2006 Gallup survey, fewer than one in three American workers strongly agreed that they had received any praise from a supervisor in the past seven days (Robison, 2006). This is concerning, as the same survey also revealed that employees who reported that they are not adequately recognized at work were three times more likely to say they would resign in the next year.

A rewards and recognition committee (or subcommittee, as the case may be) is charged with fostering an HWE by increasing rewards and recognition. Members of this committee might do the following:

- **Brainstorm reward and recognition ideas.** These could range from leaving a handwritten note in a staff member's workspace to say thank you for a job well done to putting a candy bar, a favorite snack, or some other treat in their locker or desk drawer.
- **Survey staff periodically to determine how people would like to be recognized.** Not everyone likes to be recognized by having their name announced in a busy cafeteria. Some people prefer to be recognized in private. When it comes to recognition, one size does *not* fit all.
- **Survey staff periodically to identify what types of rewards they'd like to receive.** Not every reward needs to have monetary value. You'd be surprised how many people are just as happy with verbal or written kudos as they are with a $5 meal voucher!

The committee could then disseminate the aggregate data (quarterly or biannually) to managers, supervisors, and anyone who wants to receive it. This report would not only remind and encourage leaders to recognize staff for doing good work but also provide them with ideas on how to do it.

This committee could also be responsible for placing recognition boxes with comment cards throughout the hospital and monitoring them. The cards could be printed with something as simple as, "I caught [insert name] doing [insert act], and this should be recognized." Staff could fill out these cards and place them in the box. Then, on some regular basis—say, weekly or monthly—committee members could share these cards with leadership, who could then inform staff members that they were recognized. (Again, the committee can provide ideas on how and when to do this—e.g., opening every staff meeting by acknowledging someone who was recognized or simply sending them a congratulatory email.)

> Having a rewards and recognition committee empowers staff to speak up when they see good work done—especially when formal leaders may not.

Hiring Right

This committee is responsible for educating others on best hiring practices. Most importantly, this means reminding hiring managers that they shouldn't hire based only on clinical or technical skills; they should also look for leadership skills, team-building skills, and other soft skills.

Committee members should also promote the use of behavioral-based interviewing (BBI) by hiring managers. BBI is built on the idea that a person's past performance is the best predictor of their future performance. During a BBI interview, the interviewer asks the candidate to describe specific events she has experienced, action steps she took during the event, and the successful outcome of the event. This limits the ability of the interviewee to make up stories during the interview (Byham, 2004).

Using the STAR Acronym With BBI

When conducting BBI interviews, you can use something called the STAR acronym (Byham, 2004). STAR stands for:

- **Situation:** Ask the interviewee to describe the situation—who, what, where, when, how.
- **Task:** Prompt the interviewee to describe what tasks they performed. (Note that in some cases, the situation and task may be the same.)
- **Action:** Encourage the interviewee to describe the actions they took to contribute to a successful outcome.
- **Result:** Ask the interviewee to describe the result of the efforts—preferably some type of quantifiable outcome.

For example, suppose you ask the interviewee to recount a time when they handled a patient complaint. An example of a STAR-based answer might be as follows:

- **Situation:** "I once had a patient complain about the noise level on our unit. I apologized for the noise level and thanked him for bringing the issue to my attention. Then I offered him earplugs. I also observed that this wasn't the first time a patient had complained about noise and told the patient that I would speak to my manager about looking into more effective ways to reduce noise over the long haul."
- **Task:** "With my manager's approval, I researched what other hospitals were doing to reduce noise levels."
- **Action:** "I launched a new committee, called the Pin Drop Committee, to work on ways to reduce noise based on the literature and on our own ideas."
- **Result:** "Within a few weeks after our first committee meeting, we were able to decrease overhead paging and move to more cellphone usage, as well as implement quiet hours in the afternoon in which staff had to whisper and dim lights in certain areas.
Although this outcome didn't help the patient who had lodged the initial complaint, he did express gratitude that I cared."

Finally, members of this committee should attend departmental interviews. Typically, interviews are done using a silo approach, where departmental leaders only ask other members of the department to interview a candidate (if they ask anyone at all). Rarely do you see, say, a lab associate sit in on a respiratory therapist candidate's interview. Having committee members from other departments attend departmental interviews helps build interdepartmental camaraderie while also providing everyone with insight into the hiring process.

Transformational Rounding

Rounding provides a vehicle for leaders to ask questions that help build relationships with staff (Studer, 2004). Rounding also enables leaders to act as role models and mentors, assess employee morale, harvest wins, and identify and remove barriers that prevent staff from doing their jobs. The transformational rounding committee assists in developing rounding questions for organization-wide, intradepartmental, and interdepartmental rounding, or check-ins. It also helps design rounding tools for executive leadership, managers or supervisors, nurses, and more. (See Appendix A, "Sample Rounding Template," for helpful rounding questions and tools.)

Discharge Follow-Up

Many healthcare organizations make follow-up phone calls to discharged patients. The purpose of these calls—which should be made within 48 to 72 hours of discharge—is twofold:

- **Clinical follow-up:** During the follow-up phone call, the caller should ask the patient about their condition and discuss follow-up appointments, the treatment plan, and medications and potential side effects.
- **Assessment of service:** The follow-up call can help the caller assess the patient's perception of their hospital or outpatient experience, recognize caregivers who gave excellent service, and identify areas for improvement.

To facilitate effective follow-up calls, this committee should:

- Work with individual departments to determine who will conduct the calls.
- Help departments develop scripts to guide callers in asking appropriate questions.
- Help develop an algorithm to determine whether another follow-up call, from a clinician, may be indicated.
- Track responses when patients identify areas for improvements and work with leadership, and perhaps the performance-improvement department (or other appropriate departments), to make suggestions for action plans.

Welcoming New Recruits

Retaining first-year employees is often quite difficult (Studer, 2004; Tourangeau et al., 2010). Having a welcome committee can help organizations with this effort. Members of this committee can do the following:

- Round with staff on a consistent basis during their first year of employment.

- Develop questions for each rounding session to assess the development of newly hired staff, help them adjust to the organization, solicit suggestions to improve the orientation experience, and offer help in finding resources and support.
- Regularly evaluate these questions to ensure they are obtaining the most comprehensive information.
- Act as mentors to newly hired staff, with regular meetings—perhaps biweekly at first; after 30, 60, and 90 days; after six months; and so on.

Leadership Training and Education

This committee is responsible for developing content to deliver comprehensive knowledge, skills, and education to aspiring and seasoned leaders. It plans and coordinates training, orientation, and leadership development for leaders at all levels across the organization.

Senior leadership and human resources must approve and support this committee's education and training initiatives—otherwise, the committee will lack credibility. If no such approval or support is forthcoming, the committee could still exist as a journal club, with committee members sharing published and evidence-based leadership research and outcomes at various departmental staff meetings.

Physician and Staff Engagement

Physician engagement and staff engagement are key drivers to the success of any healthcare organization. To promote engagement, I suggest forming not one, but two committees: one for physician engagement and one for staff engagement.

The physician engagement committee could meet on a regular basis with senior leaders to discuss important topics like goal-setting, patient safety, and leadership development.

Members of this committee could also introduce new programs and projects to the medical staff. Finally, the committee could incorporate physician practice managers in medical staff meetings and establish teams composed of board, management, and physicians to weigh in on key decisions, leadership development, peer review, and so forth.

As for the staff engagement committee, its duties might include the following:

- Working closely with the rewards and recognition committee to support its efforts
- Reviewing staff satisfaction surveys to identify commonalities and areas for improvements on an organizational level

- Organizing engagement activities, such as celebrations and potluck meals, and assisting in selecting gifts for employees—for example, to commemorate their work anniversary or mark other occasions or accomplishments

Bright Ideas

The main mission of this committee (which may in fact be a subcommittee of a larger project improvement committee) is to surface suggestions from staff for workplace improvements—for example, by placing Bright Idea boxes with comment cards throughout the organization or by offering a dedicated suggestion form on the organization's website.

Of course, it's not enough to simply solicit suggestions from staff. This committee should also have a process in place to evaluate suggestions and implement those that can bring about positive change. If staff offer dozens of ideas but none are acted upon, the flow of suggestions will wither and die—along with the attitude and trust of the staff.

Finally, this committee can develop and launch special programs related to areas such as safety, cost reduction, or patient and staff satisfaction. On the safety side, the committee might implement safety huddles and encourage units to use briefings, debriefings, and other huddles to improve interdepartmental communication. These methods and other tools in the TeamSTEPPS program can be used to create a culture of safety and transparency.

> TeamSTEPPS is an evidence-based system designed for use in clinical practice to optimize patient outcomes by improving communication and teamwork (Agency for Healthcare Research and Quality, n.d.).

Motivating Others to Obtain Buy-In

Any initiative to promote an HWE needs buy-in from hospital staff. That means motivating them to take part in the initiative. Simply put, motivating others is about engaging them to behave in a way that achieves a specific and immediate goal (Brady & Cummings, 2010). It's the art and talent of moving people to act in a way that achieves a desired change or outcome.

Witt (n.d.) provides a few tips on how to motivate others:

- **Be specific.** Explain what the goal is and discuss what the other person's role would be in achieving it. Don't be abstract—for example, don't say, "I want everyone to do their best." Instead, spell out the goal using the SMART technique. SMART is a goal-setting acronym that helps us to develop goals that are:
    - Specific
    - Measurable

- **A**ttainable
- **R**ealistic
- **T**imely

- **Be timely.** It's easier to ask people to commit to a specific time frame than to expect them to meet indefinitely. Set a start date and an end date.
- **Roll up your sleeves.** Real leaders wouldn't ask someone to do something they wouldn't do themselves. In other words, don't instruct staff to work on a project and then walk away from it. Share the load in some way so the group doesn't feel neglected.
- **Look in the mirror.** People are motivated by positive emotions like excitement, pride, and joy. Don't expect others to exhibit these emotions if you don't.
- **Inspire.** Using a "what's in it for me" approach, offer multiple and specific reasons why you are asking for their participation.

> Even members of an organization who do not have a formal leadership role can work to motivate others. The positive results of this type of effort have an added benefit—a dose of dopamine, the neurotransmitter that stimulates positive feelings and decreases frustration, depression, anger, and anxiety.

Motivating others is not a one-time effort. It must be sustained. All too often, change initiatives fail not because people weren't good at motivating others to join in at the beginning but because efforts to motivate people weren't sustained throughout the life of the initiative.

Promoting Transformational Leadership

Transformational leadership is a leadership style in which leaders create HWEs, in which employees feel motivated, supported, and encouraged to be creative and take risks. This leadership style is often seen in Magnet®-designated hospitals (Ulrich et al., 2009).

Characteristics of the positive environment associated with transformational leadership include the following (Salanova et al., 2011):

- Shared goals, values, and missions
- Distributed power
- Education
- Behavior modeling
- Individualized guidance
- Open, effective communication

Transformational leadership stands in contrast to transactional leadership (MacGregor Burns, 1978). *Transactional leadership* involves an exchange relationship—a transaction between leaders and followers. In this transaction, followers typically receive financial compensation in exchange for complying with a leader's request. In contrast, transformational leadership empowers employees to go above and beyond to achieve organizational goals—for example, by improving a process that makes a positive impact on overall organizational excellence.

Bernard Bass (1985) identified subcomponents of transformational leadership, including the following:

- **Idealized influence:** Transformational leaders act as role models for staff. They are respected, admired, and trusted by their followers because they consistently do the right thing and exhibit high moral and ethical standards. (Note that Bass originally referred to this subcomponent of transformational leadership as *charisma*.)
- **Inspirational motivation:** Transformational leaders show enthusiasm and optimism as they motivate others to commit to a shared vision and shared goals.
- **Intellectual stimulation:** Transformational leaders encourage creativity and inspire followers to think about old problems in new ways.
- **Individualized consideration:** Transformational leaders respect the needs and desires of others and accept their differences. Because followers feel worthwhile and gain a sense of purpose, they continuously develop higher levels of potential.

Casida and Parker (2011) suggest that training in transformational leadership should be a foundational requirement of nursing managers. Indeed, they argue that it is a moral obligation of administrators to place competent transformational leaders into formal leadership roles. Yet, many people who hold formal leadership titles are selected for their roles due to their seniority, their clinical proficiency, their technical abilities, or simply the need to fill the position (Sherman et al., 2007). Therefore, they lack transformational leadership skills.

Fortunately, training in transformational leadership is available. This training can consist of formal leadership classes, courses, and lectures; online and continuing education activities; and journal readings. One excellent resource is offered jointly by the American Organization of Nurse Executives, the Association of Perioperative Registered Nurses, and the American Association of Critical-Care Nurses to assist current and emerging nurse leaders in obtaining necessary leadership competencies (Sherman & Pross, 2010).

Just because a nurse has clinical expertise does not mean they also possesses leadership skills. Even nurses with informal leadership abilities often struggle to employ these in their new formal role. Without leadership training, many new nurse leaders become frustrated and fail (Sherman & Pross, 2010). Remember: In the words of Sherman and Pross (2010, para. 11), "The development of leadership skills should be viewed as a journey."

Accountability Versus Ownership

One key way to foster an HWE is to encourage our colleagues not just to be accountable but to become "owners" of the organization. To grasp the difference between ownership and accountability, consider the way you behave in a hotel versus how you behave at home. For example, in a hotel room, I hold myself accountable for the condition of the room to the extent that I try to keep things relatively tidy and throw away any trash. But that's as far as it goes. I don't make the bed, I leave my used towels on the floor for housekeeping to wash them, and so on. At home, however, I clean constantly. I make the bed. I wash the towels and rehang them. I haul my trash outside. That's because I have ownership of my home. Simply put, the success and future of any organization is directly related to the care everyone there provides to both patients and colleagues. Staff who feel a sense of ownership offer better care.

Staff engagement is a key driver of this sense of ownership. Engaged staff deliver higher quality of care than mediocre or disgruntled staff. Engaged staff can also help their organization attract and retain patients and families. An important part of engagement is loyalty. This includes staff loyalty, which is often demonstrated through quality of care; patient and family loyalty, which drives them to choose your organization over any others; and loyalty among formal and informal leaders, which fosters trusting relationships.

The Drive Home

Let's drive home the key points in this chapter:

- An HWE provides staff with a feeling of inclusion, safety, and motivation.
- Change leadership is a key part of sustaining an HWE.
- Changing behavior is one of the biggest challenges organizations face. According to LaClair and Rao (2002), roughly 70% of all changes in all organizations fail.
- Even though 70% of changes fail, you can succeed if you overcome cynicism and fear, lack of applied knowledge, and lack of practiced skills. Identify hidden conflicts that undermine your efforts, and know the unwritten rules that work against change.

- Sustaining HWEs must be a priority if healthcare organizations want to make meaningful contributions in the care of patients and patients' families.
- Patient safety is the top priority—always.
- Take a risk and start a committee to improve your workplace environment.
- Recognition for doing good work releases dopamine in the brain, which creates feelings of pride and pleasure.
- All leaders, formal and informal, are responsible for keeping healthcare providers engaged in providing patient-centered care.
- To motivate others, we need to be specific, timely, participative, active, and inspiring.
- Transformational leadership is an optimal leadership style in which leaders create environments in which employees are motivated, supported, and encouraged to be creative and take risks.
- Encourage your colleagues to become "owners" of the organization.

References

Agency for Healthcare Research and Quality. (n.d.). *TeamSTEPPS*. http://teamstepps.ahrq.gov

American Association of Critical-Care Nurses. (2016). *AACN standards for establishing and sustaining healthy work environments: A journey to excellence* (2nd ed.). https://www.aacn.org/wd/hwe/docs/hwestandards.pdf

Bass, B. M. (1985). *Leadership and performance beyond expectations*. Free Press.

Blake, N. (2016). Barriers to implementing and sustaining healthy work environments. *AACN Advanced Critical Care, 27*(1), 21-23. https://doi.org/10.4037/aacnacc2016553

Brady, G. P., & Cummings, G. G. (2010). The influence of nursing leadership on nurse performance: A systematic literature review. *Journal of Nursing Management, 18*(4), 425–439. https://doi.org/10.1111/j.1365-2834.2010.01100.x

Brunges, M., & Foley-Brinza, C. (2014). Projects for increasing job satisfaction and creating a healthy work environment. *AORN Journal, 100*(6), 670–681. https://doi.org/10.1016/j.aorn.2014.01.029

Byham, W. C. (2004). *Targeted selection: A behavioral approach to improved hiring decisions*. Development Dimensions International.

Casida, J., & Parker, J. (2011). Staff nurse perceptions of nurse manager leadership styles and outcomes. *Journal of Nursing Management, 19*(4), 478–486. https://doi.org/10.1111/j.1365-2834.2011.01252.x

Cowden, T., Cummings, G., & Profetto-McGrath, J. (2011). Leadership practices and staff nurses' intent to stay: A systematic review. *Journal of Nursing Management, 19*(4), 461–477. https://doi.org/10.1111/j.1365-2834.2011.01209.x

Cummings, G. G., MacGregor, T., Davey, M., Lee, H., Wong, C. A., Lo, E., Muise, M., & Stafford, E. (2010). Leadership styles and outcome patterns for the nursing workforce and work environment: A systematic review. *International Journal of Nursing Studies, 47*(3), 363–385. https://doi.org/10.1016/j.ijnurstu.2009.08.006

Geedey, N. (2006). Create and sustain a healthy work environment. *Nursing Management, 37*(10), 17–18.

Kelly, L. A., Wicker, T. L., & Gerkin, R. D. (2014). The relationship of training and education to leadership practices in frontline nurse leaders. *Journal of Nursing Administration, 44*(3), 158-163. https://doi.org/10.1097/NNA.0000000000000044

LaClair, J. A., & Rao, R. P. (2002, Nov. 1). Helping employees embrace change. *McKinsey Quarterly*. https://www.mckinsey.com/capabilities/people-and-organizational-performance/our-insights/helping-employees-embrace-change

MacGregor Burns, J. (1978). *Leadership*. Harper and Row.

Meyer, P. J. (2003). *Attitude is everything! If you want to succeed above and beyond!* Meyer Resource Group, Inc.

Pund, L. E., & Sklar, P. (2012). *Linking quality assurance to human resources: Improving patient satisfaction by improving employee satisfaction*. Indiana University School of Public and Environmental Affairs. https://spea.sitehost.iu.edu/pubs/undergrad-honors/volumn-6/Pund,%20Lindsey%20-%20Linking%20Quality%20Assurance%20to%20Human%20Resources%20Improving%20Patient%20Satisfaction%20by%20Improving%20Employee%20Satisfaction%20-%20Faculty%20Pam%20Sklar.pdf

Robison, J. (2006, Nov. 9). *In praise of praising your employees*. Gallup. https://www.gallup.com/workplace/236951/praise-praising-employees.aspx

Salanova, M., Lorente, L., Chambel, M. J., & Martínez, I. M. (2011). Linking transformational leadership to nurses' extra-role performance: The mediating role of self-efficacy and work engagement. *Journal of Advanced Nursing, 67*(10), 2256–2266. https://doi.org/10.1111/j.1365-2648.2011.05652.x

Sherman, R. O., Bishop, M., Eggenberger, T., & Karden, R. (2007). Development of a leadership competency model. *Journal of Nursing Administration, 37*(2), 85–94. https://doi.org/10.1097/00005110-200702000-00011

Sherman, R., & Pross, E. (2010). Growing future nurse leaders to build and sustain healthy work environments at the unit level. *The Online Journal of Issues in Nursing, 15*(1). https://doi.org/10.3912/OJIN.Vol15No01Man01

Smith, M. K. (2005). *Bruce W. Tuckman—forming, storming, norming and performing in groups*. infed. http://infed.org/mobi/bruce-w-tuckman-forming-storming-norming-and-performing-in-groups/

Studer, Q. (2004). *Hardwiring excellence: Purpose, worthwhile work, making a difference*. Studer Fire Starter Publishing.

Tourangeau, A. E., Cummings, G., Cranley, L. A., Ferron, E. M., & Harvey, S. (2010). Determinants of hospital nurse intention to remain employed: Broadening our understanding. *Journal of Advanced Nursing, 66*(1), 22–32. https://doi.org/10.1111/j.1365-2648.2009.05190.x

Tuckman, B. W. (1965). Developmental sequence in small groups. *Psychological Bulletin, 63*(6), 384–399. https://doi.org/10.1037/h0022100

Ulrich, B. T., Buerhaus, P. I., Donelan, K., Norman, L., & Dittus, R. (2009). Magnet status and registered nurse views of the work environment and nursing as a career. *Journal of Nursing Administration, 39*(7-8), S54–S62. https://doi.org/10.1097/01.NNA.0000269745.24889.c6

Witt, C. (n.d.). *How to motivate and inspire your people in difficult times*. Reliable Plant. http://www.reliableplant.com/Read/18525/how-to-motivate-inspire-your-people-in-difficult-times

10
Organizational Culture and Behavior

Shelley Johnson (Chapter Contributor)

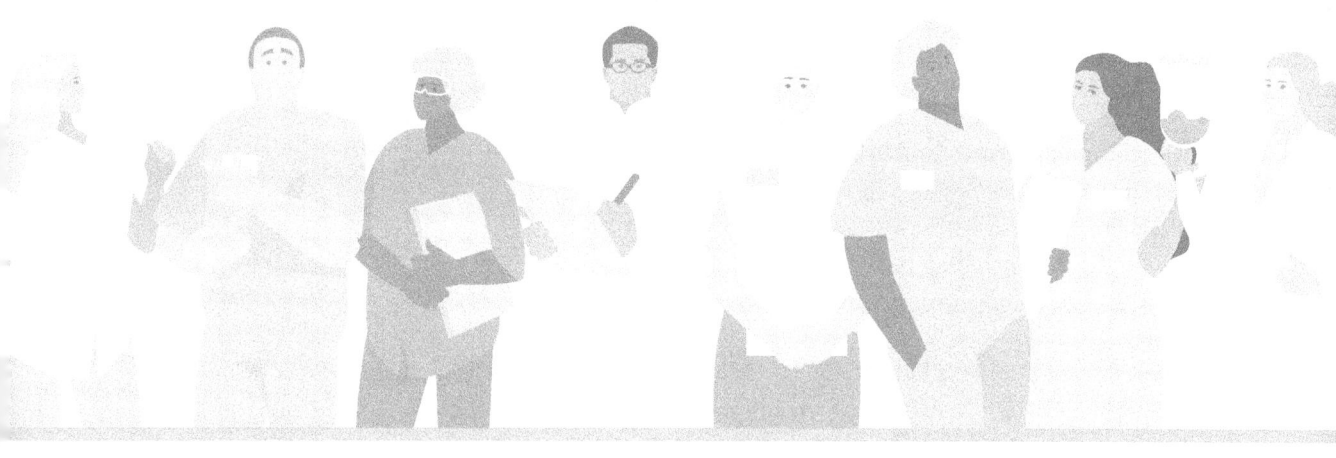

"We are what we repeatedly do."
–Will Durant

This chapter takes a closer look at communication in the context of organizational culture and behavior. More specifically, it discusses how your role as an effective communicator contributes to the organizational culture and climate on a micro and macro level. As you read this chapter, reflect on your work environments—past and present—and consider how both you and your colleagues have contributed to the organizational culture and climate through direct intentional acts or through acts of omission as they relate to communication.

In the Driver's Seat: Defining Organizational Culture and Behavior

By itself, *culture* refers to characteristics historically shared by a group of people that are self-determined or defined by outsiders looking in. Everyone belongs to numerous cultures and subcultures. Because people are so complex and culturally integrated, attempts to neatly place individuals into distinct categories when working toward organizational progress are both impractical and ineffective. In contrast, *organizational culture* can be defined by all the life experiences, strengths, weaknesses, education, upbringing, and so forth of an organization's executives and employees. As for *cultural behavior,* it describes one aspect of social traditions used to shape environmental and group values. It pertains to how people and groups in organizations behave. It also considers the role of organizational systems, structures, and processes in shaping behavior to understand how organizations really work.

Organizational culture and behavior have a direct effect on efficiency, patient outcomes, patient experience, and the financial bottom line. A positive culture begets positive outcomes, including staff engagement, fair-mindedness, energy, team spirit, and inventiveness.

> Although executive leaders play a significant role in defining organizational culture through their actions and leadership, all employees contribute to the organizational culture.

Every organizational culture has both visible and invisible values. Examples of visible values may include symbols, customs, formalities, language, structures, clothing, technology, and history. Invisible values include beliefs, decision-making trends, administrative support (or lack thereof), rules, procedures, and responses to change.

Here are a few examples of healthcare organizations that are known for their strong organizational culture and how they accomplished this:

- **Mayo Clinic:** This renowned nonprofit medical group and research institution is widely recognized for its patient-centered culture. The organization places a strong emphasis on collaboration, teamwork, and continuous learning among its staff, resulting in high-quality care and positive patient experiences.

- **Cleveland Clinic:** This leading academic medical center is known for its culture of excellence and innovation. The organization values a patient-first approach and fosters a culture of empathy, compassion, and personalized care. Cleveland Clinic also emphasizes continuous improvement and encourages its employees to contribute to research and advancements in healthcare.
- **Kaiser Permanente:** A large integrated healthcare delivery system that places a strong focus on preventive care and wellness. The organization's culture promotes patient engagement, teamwork, and a commitment to delivering affordable, high-quality care. Kaiser Permanente also emphasizes the importance of diversity, equity, and inclusion in its organizational culture.
- **Geisinger Health System:** Geisinger is an integrated health services organization known for its commitment to patient-centered care and innovation. The organization has implemented a unique ProvenCare model that focuses on evidence-based practices and continuous improvement. Geisinger fosters a culture of transparency, collaboration, and accountability among its employees.
- **Studer Group:** Although not a healthcare provider itself, Studer Group is a consultancy firm that specializes in helping healthcare organizations improve their organizational culture and performance. They work with various healthcare institutions to develop and implement strategies that enhance employee engagement, patient satisfaction, and overall organizational effectiveness.

I have worked in small and large organizations among racially and ethnically homogenous and heterogeneous groups. What I have gleaned from these experiences is that organizational culture and behavior have less to do with race and ethnicity than they do with the distribution of power and control. This in turn influences communication within the organization.

Most nurses seek a clear-cut methodology for making decisions and taking action. However, a fear of failure can stifle our potentially courageous attempts at doing what we consider correct, especially as it relates to organizational culture. Often, an organization's culture can lure us into doing things the way they've always been done to stay within the organization's norms—even though we know it's not the best choice. That was the case for a small rural hospital that had a labor and delivery unit, a postpartum unit, a pediatric unit, and a newborn nursery, each with its own nurse manager. Because these nurse managers were considered the clinical experts on their unit, the normal procedure was for staff to forward all problems to the respective nurse manager and let her solve them.

Hospital administrators decided to reorganize the nursing management structure among these departments. They appointed one nurse manager as the maternal-child director and placed the other three nurse managers into clinical coordinator roles. However, this organizational change made it difficult for the new director to gather all the necessary facts regarding all the different units to make the best decisions.

The staff criticized the director for poor decisions she made due to her lack of clinical expertise in the other nurse managers' specialties. The director recognized her weaknesses in these areas but did not admit this to her staff for fear it would make her appear even less capable. And because she had been responsible for solving problems in her unit in the past, she continued to try to independently resolve issues that arose instead of allowing the clinical coordinators or frontline staff to help. Subsequently, many seasoned nurses resigned.

> **Time to Reflect**
>
> Reflect on your work experiences. Does your organization's culture affect how forthcoming you are when addressing issues with colleagues, patients, and/or administration? Why or why not?

What does all this have to do with organizational culture? Simple: This healthcare facility had an organizational culture that emphasized cost control over care—indicated by its decision to reorganize the nursing management structure. It's no surprise it found itself unable to retain staff.

Successful Cultural Behaviors

Successful organizations share many common cultural behaviors. These include the following:

- Providing employment security
- Engaging in selective hiring
- Using self-managed teams
- Being decentralized
- Paying well
- Training employees
- Reducing status differences
- Embracing transparency

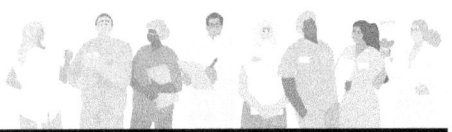

The Importance of Cultural Behaviors

When are cultural behaviors important? ALWAYS! This includes scenarios that involve the following:

- Forming and maintaining relationships with patients and colleagues
- Interacting with patients and colleagues
- Opposite gender interactions
- Like gender interactions
- Interactions between members of the same generation or different generations
- Interactions between members of races that are similar or different

Your Road Map: Understanding Organizational Cultural and Behaviors

The behaviors of those you work with can help you gain a better understanding of an organization's culture. These behaviors often relate to the following:

- Power and control
- Adaptation or deception
- Etiquette
- Formality
- Perception of time
- Hierarchy and gender
- Communication
- Cliques and work ethic

> Organizational culture is often enduring—but it can change. For example, it may be that an organization did not always tolerate this type of behavior, but the current climate does. This is often a result of leaders who tolerate certain behaviors from employees.

Power and Control

In nursing, the concepts of power and control normally have negative connotations. Nurses' aversion to the overt quest for power stems from our cultural indoctrination, which emphasizes humility, self-sacrifice, and servant leadership. As a result, nurses often employ other tactics to assert power and control, such as passive aggression, a lack of transparency, and negative competition practices. Often, desperation fuels our need for control.

You've probably encountered frontline staff who operate like this. Maybe it was a receptionist who made you wait 10 minutes before acknowledging your presence. Or maybe it was a telephone operator who put you on hold for an extended period and then demanded that you explain what you needed so she could discuss it with the person you were trying to talk to. This type of behavior positions you as a victim of the organization's culture and behaviors, informs you of who is holding the power, and reveals how control is exercised.

In both examples, it's obvious these employees have been given an inappropriate level of power and control, based on their communication style. Specifically, they have too much power, and it's being abused. To remedy this situation, they need training in customer service and a better management team to coach them.

Adaptation or Deception

As professionals, we like to think of ourselves as consistent. After all, consistency has a very positive connotation. We equate consistency with honesty, trust, transparency, and authenticity. The truth is, however, that consistency is unnatural. We all operate within multiple cultures—to the point where we often switch cultural personae from one moment to another based on our environment.

Given this reality, it's fair to say that consistency is often the opposite of honesty, transparency, and authenticity. Indeed, it can even be a form of dishonesty. I discovered this during my teen years, during which I attended a very suburban, affluent, Caucasian, fundamentalist Christian high school but lived and worshipped in an area populated with immigrants and other minority groups. I quickly learned that I had to become a chameleon of sorts—adapting my persona to successfully integrate into the varied settings in which I found myself. Of course, this is not to say that you should lose yourself, be a fraud, or pretend. Rather, you should take the time to learn about others and do your best to respect their culture while working to preserve your own identity.

I would be a liar if I didn't admit that at times I felt like I was wearing different masks or even trying to manipulate others, or that I occasionally felt angry and resentful about what I perceived as a mandate to conform. But I also learned that a sort of cultural balance can emerge from being culturally open—that is, temporarily putting aside one's values and norms to demonstrate acceptance of other cultures and adapt to different cultural climates. Indeed, this convergence of cultures can result in the formation of new cultural norms! Not surprisingly, this goes a long way toward facilitating communication among members of these different groups.

> The assimilation of a minority into the majority's culture is often more of a defense mechanism aimed to improve chances of survival than a tool to achieve acceptance or a sincere desire to integrate.

Etiquette

Members of different cultures practice different forms of etiquette. As a result, they may be perceived differently by members of other groups. For example, African and West Indian people are known for their excessive politeness and passivity. For those who are not used to it, their constant smiles and nods can appear saccharine. I learned this firsthand. As an immigrant from a West Indian country, I was very accustomed to smiling and chatting with strangers. But while riding on Philadelphia's subway system, I quickly learned that smiling and engaging in conversation uninvited was a little like throwing a punch: More often than not, the recipients of my efforts responded with surprise and even aggression.

In business environments, a culture of politeness can contribute to poor communication. The fact that everyone is smiling and nodding should not be interpreted as agreement or support. Moreover, some people in this type of environment view disagreement as disrespectful and a challenge to those in authority.

> It is vital to learn about the etiquette used by others and not to take differences personally!

Formality

During my career I've worked in two very different healthcare settings. Healthcare setting A was a large multispecialty institution that was internationally known for its research and its awards for nursing excellence. In contrast, healthcare setting B was a small, relatively unknown rural hospital.

The employees in these settings demonstrated very different levels of formality in their communications. In healthcare setting A, nurses, doctors, and administrators addressed each other by their first names. In healthcare setting B, the common practice was to use titles at all times—such as Doctor, Nurse, and Professor for employees, and Miss, Mrs., and Mr. for patients. (Incidentally, employees at healthcare setting B also often referred to patients as "consumers.")

The lower level of formality in healthcare setting A made it appear that employees were confident in their view of themselves and their abilities, while the employees in healthcare setting B seemed to be working too hard to command respect. Their use of formality had other effects, too. For example, by rigidly enforcing a hierarchy by using titles, they effectively divided the "top" people from those on the "bottom." This resulted in an us-versus-them mentality and practice. Because of this divide, many staff adopted a submissive role. Frontline staff and even administrators often felt too cowed to speak up when they detected a potential problem. As a result, healthcare setting B always appeared to exist in a reactive state rather than a proactive one.

Perception of Time

Some cultures perceive time differently from others. For example, many Westerners are quite fixated on time, equating it with concepts such as productivity, efficiency, and finances. Members of some other cultures, however, place less importance on time—or, more specifically, punctuality.

In the beginning of my career, I worked for a nurse-run health center in a Philadelphia housing development for underserved minorities. Residents seeking care were required to make an appointment. Often, however, they arrived very late for these appointments or skipped them altogether without canceling them first. And, of course, their health conditions only continued to worsen as a result.

Everyone (including me) complained bitterly about this situation. We took it personally—like the population we were trying to serve didn't appreciate us. We even assigned negative labels to frequent offenders. I can only imagine how the population we were meant to serve regarded us. No doubt they found us pushy, condescending, sanctimonious, and egotistical!

Because we expected our hosting culture—that is, the residents of the housing development—to conform to our demands, we had unintentionally created a climate of conflict. To rectify this, we reviewed our organizational culture and identified ways we could change to better meet the needs of the community. As part of this effort, we no longer required residents to make appointments to be seen by a caregiver on certain days of the week. For those days we did take appointments, we instituted flexible appointment times, for which patients were double-booked. We also started asking patients why they missed appointments. This revealed that patients often missed appointments due to other pressing issues, which they did not feel comfortable sharing before.

The effects of these changes to the organizational culture were twofold: They increased trust and understanding between us and the community, and they increased the number of patients who came to us for care.

Hierarchy and Gender

Some healthcare environments enforce a strict hierarchical structure. In these settings, leaders are very demanding of those holding lesser titles, who are expected to be submissive. These leaders command respect but have little regard for others. These leaders frequently issue commands without service-level input. Many believe they are untouchable and unreachable—almost like demigods—and expect others to revere them. This explains why, in settings like these, you often hear statements such as, "I would never attempt to speak with the CNO directly," or, "Be willing to let your supervisors take credit for your work!"

Gender may also play a role in the organizational hierarchy. For example, in many healthcare environments, men dominate administration. Although middle management is generally balanced between males and females, women are rarely represented in upper executive management. Women are generally the controlling majority in nursing administration, however.

In my experience, organizations with a shared governance model have more effective communication—both horizontally and vertically within the hierarchy—than organizations that do not practice this model. *Shared governance* is a culturally sensitive professional practice model that emphasizes the principles of partnership, equity, and ownership to promote accountability-based decision-making. Shared governance is also an interdisciplinary approach to providing excellent patient care that offers frontline staff some power and control in decision-making (Barden et al., 2011). When the power to make decisions goes beyond administrators, staff can communicate potential or existing problems more effectively and efficiently.

Regardless of whether your organization uses a shared governance model or a more traditional hierarchical structure, there may be times when you need to direct an issue to the attention of someone other than your boss. Script 10.1 contains an example of a conversation you might have with your boss when you need to direct an issue to the attention of that person's manager.

Hierarchy in Action

Dr. Solemn, who hailed from India, had enlisted an Ivy League graduate, doctoral-prepared research fellow to work on a laboratory research project that involved the management of high-level research instruments. This research fellow happily worked night and day on the project. Indeed, many faculty and students witnessed this fellow dashing to Dr. Solemn's side, excitement evident on his face. The fellow was willing to serve and responded to every command and request with urgency.

One day, an American visitor came to the facility. While standing in a corridor with Dr. Solemn, the visitor saw him make a subtle gesture at the research fellow down the hall. The fellow broke into a sprint toward Dr. Solemn, as if drawn by a powerful magnet. "There's no need for you to run!" the visitor cried in an attempt to be friendly. Dr. Solemn immediately turned to the visitor and said, "It is necessary, as I am his senior."

The moral of this story? Members of different cultures show—and expect to receive—respect in different ways.

SCRIPT 10.1

What to say when…

YOU FEEL YOU NEED TO GO ABOVE YOUR NURSE MANAGER.

T
Time and place to talk

Choose an appropriate time and place to have a conversation with your supervisor. Find a quiet and private setting where you can discuss the issue without interruptions.

Example: Nurse Manager

> *(After repeated conversations on nurse-patient ratios) Jeff, I know it feels like we've exhausted the staffing issues on our unit; however, I feel the need to continue to pursue this issue. When is a good time to meet?*

E
Explain and explore perspectives

Clearly and calmly explain the situation to your supervisor, providing specific details about how someone else took credit for your work. Be objective and stick to the facts.

> *We are placing our patients in jeopardy of unsafe care. I appreciate your listening to my concerns in the past, yet my concerns still remain strong. I'd like to speak with Greg [Jeff's manager] to see if he has any other suggestions, and I welcome you joining me in this meeting. How does that sound?*

L
Listen to their perspective

Allow your supervisor to share their thoughts and gather their perspective on the situation. Listen actively and be open to their feedback or insights.

Example A: Receptive

> *OK, I will schedule a meeting, but just so you know, I did already present this, and Greg didn't seem to think it was such an issue.*

> *I appreciate that you already addressed this, but I am eager to give my own personal angle on this. I think it's important that your manager sees from all of us just how important the issue is.*

Example B: Defensive

> *There is no reason to beat a dead horse on this issue. I already spoke to Greg about this.*

I appreciate that you already addressed this, but I am eager to give my own personal angle on this. I think it's important that Greg considers my point of view too.

L
Leverage shared values and lead the conversation forward

Remind your supervisor of the shared goals and values within the workplace, such as fairness, recognition, and teamwork. Emphasize the importance of accurate recognition and the impact it has on the overall work environment.

Example A: Receptive

> *I'm anxious to hear if Greg tells you the same thing he told me.*

I will explain to Greg that you have been very receptive in listening to my concerns. And I will explain that I called this meeting because this issue is incredibly important to me, and I really wanted to speak personally about this.

Example B: Unreceptive

> *Greg will be angry that you're wasting his time!*

Respectfully, I would still like to meet with him. It is important to me that I share this information and do what is right to advocate for the safety of our patients.

Communication

Children of every culture have been on the receiving end of "mom eyes," otherwise known as "the look." This penetrating glare delivers a telepathic scolding. Similarly, supervisors in organizations use body language to encourage or deter behaviors among employees. As adults, we like to believe we are beyond this type of basic conditioning, but another person's tone, body position, subtle eye movements, and grunts can cause us to close our mouths and bend our heads in shame.

Nonverbal scolding is just one type of communication. Another is the exchange of information. Information is valuable, and communicating it on any level exposes all people participating in the exchange in various ways. Knowledge can be both a power and a threat. Information control is a well-known method to intimidate, sabotage, and manipulate others. In a work setting, when you demonstrate that you have more information than your leaders, you will remain valuable only until you have no further information to share—or until they begin to perceive you as the competition.

Of course, the words we choose have a profound effect on our communications. They can be used to build or destroy. For example, consider that some healthcare organizations refer to clients as patients, while others call them consumers. This changes the context: A patient is perceived as someone who *seeks* care, while a consumer is someone who *buys* care. Similarly, supervisors who refer to personnel as workers instead of colleagues imply that they are valued more for their ability to complete tasks than for their contributions to planning and managing care.

All this is to say that different healthcare organizations have different ways of communicating. For example, some organizations embrace differences of opinion, while others may frown on employees who don't automatically say "yes." In addition, there are overt ways of communicating within the organization as well as covert ways. All this plays into the organization's broader culture.

Cliques and Work Ethic

Movies often portray high school kids as existing within a social hierarchy. This hierarchy often consists of cliques that contain nerds (known as very diligent students), athletes (respected for their looks and physical abilities), or cool kids (who are popular, often wealthy, self-centered, and sometimes mean). Most modern teen-targeted movies glorify another clique, however: the cool slackers—kids who appear not to try too hard.

Sadly, this same clique seems to dominate in the workplace. This explains why you may sometimes hear unit banter along the lines of, "Ugh, why does Alicia always try to be Superwoman? She tries too hard! She must *really* want to be liked. Why else would she pretend to be so motivated?" Obviously, comments like these don't convey collegiality. Instead, they ooze envy, malice, and bullying.

When behaviors like these become part of the culture, the result is an unhealthy workplace. I observed this firsthand some years ago when I worked at a small hospital as one of three nurse managers. One of the other nurse managers was extremely professional, positive, and friendly. Rather than embracing these excellent qualities, hospital employees took any chance they could to complain or make sarcastic comments about my upbeat and motivated partner.

In addition to affecting employee behavior, organizational culture has a direct effect on work ethic. The work ethic of an organization is generally set by administrators. To promote a positive work ethic, leaders must intentionally model productivity, balance, strategic risk-taking, and a willingness to grow and develop. Having a positive work ethic doesn't mean doing all the work, however. It's certainly appropriate for leaders to delegate tasks—but only if those tasks fit the employee's job description.

EMBRACE and ACCEPT to Improve Cultural Awareness

To improve your cultural awareness, you can EMBRACE and ACCEPT culture.

EMBRACE:

Encourage openness and discussion.

Model standards of behavior.

Be still and observe.

Reflect on the accuracy of assumptions and stereotypes.

Ask questions to seek clarification.

Consider how you present yourself.

Engage with others and become an active participant in learning.

ACCEPT:

Acknowledge that differences exist.

Consider others.

Celebrate diversity.

Empathize.

Perceive the environment.

Tolerate only respect.

What Drives People

Social acceptance drives people to some degree. But it's not the only thing. Other motivators, such as service, collaboration, and the achievement of personal goals, are central driving forces for many people.

I once read an article that equated work with happiness—but not because the work produced financial gain or recognition (McKee, 2017). Instead, it was because staff felt a sense of satisfaction from a job well done. Simply put, productive work is important!

I have found that employees rarely complain about work assignments or overload when they feel competent and valued. Feelings of self-worth, purpose, and dignity abound from a job well done.

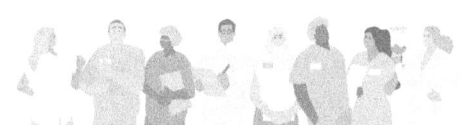

Assessing and Improving Organizational Culture and Behavior

In the words of Traphagan (2017), culture is complex. Before you can improve organizational culture and behaviors, you must assess these facets of your organization. Consider the following:

- What ideas and beliefs do people at the top of the organizational hierarchy hold as true and inviolate?
- How do your colleagues feel about sharing their ideas among themselves and with formal leaders?
- How are employees evaluated, and how are promotions given?
- What is the organization's image in the community?
- What does it take to implement change?

The answers to these questions will provide direction for improvement.

Improving organizational culture and behavior is no easy task. Influencing and energizing members of the organization to follow a shared vision can be challenging! Organizational leaders must model and support a positive culture as it relates to social interactions, communication, shared interests and responsibilities, collaboration, and friendships. Of course, formal leaders can influence organizational culture—shaping and molding the values, basic assumptions, and beliefs shared by the members of the organization. But informal leaders can also play a key role in ensuring that the organizational culture supports good relationships that empower everyone in their work. The integrity of the informal leadership of the organization is just as critical as that of the formal leaders.

One crucial aspect of fostering the desired organizational culture and behaviors is to show respect. This includes showing respect for the cultural and ethnic backgrounds of all families and colleagues. It also includes making yourself accessible to others and demonstrating a willingness to focus on their concerns.

Another way to show respect is to become aware of the following:

- Behaviors exhibited and accepted by members of the organization when they interact, such as the language they use, any rituals they follow, and their general demeanor
- Norms or standards that develop in working groups
- Collective beliefs about what is important—in other words, values supported by the organization—such as quality, diversity, inclusion, and collaboration
- Philosophies that guide policies and procedures
- Rules and customs in the organization
- How others perceive different organizational practices

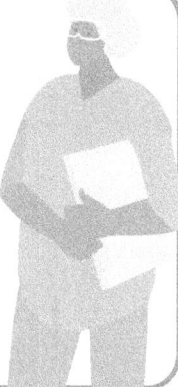

Time to Reflect

Consider how changes in your organization are communicated both externally and internally. How might these internal and external communications be improved?

Showing respect is just one way to improve organizational culture and behaviors. Other ways through which improved organizational culture and behaviors come about include the following:

- **Organizational changes:** Organizations are dynamic in nature—constantly shifting in response to external changes (e.g., healthcare reform) and internal changes (e.g., employee turnover). This constant change forces organizations into a continual state of learning and developing, which results in new perspectives. These new perspectives must be communicated and embraced by members of the organization (Watkins, 2013).
- **Enculturation:** This is a socialization process by which healthcare professionals adjust to and become part of the culture of a new hospital, office, department, unit, etc. Some organizations help new employees enculturate through orientation or onboarding sessions and other human

In addition to helping socialize healthcare professionals in a new position or organization, enculturation can serve to initiate change (Pfeffer & Veiga, 1999). For example, the CNO at one workplace of mine attended each new nurse orientation session not only to welcome all new recruits but also to urge them to challenge processes that didn't make sense and to share with her suggestions for improvement. Her remarks granted us permission to communicate our thoughts and ideas—and to drive change.

resources initiatives such as mentoring programs. (Chapter 9 discusses mentoring programs in more detail.)

- **Fostering trust:** The best way to promote positive enculturation is by providing a trusting work environment. Fostering trust means telling the truth to leadership colleagues, patients, and families, even when it is difficult. It means being authentic and trustworthy in your dealings with others. Finally, it means being transparent about the thought process and background behind important decisions.

- **Sharing stories to inspire others:** Share stories about the workplace that reinforce the organizational culture you seek to achieve and that recognize positive behaviors and characteristics among you and your colleagues. The tone and content of these stories are powerful forces in shaping and strengthening your work climate and frequently become imprinted on the organizational mind.

> Try listening—really listening—to the stories your colleagues share. Are they inspiring stories—say, about that time the healthcare team worked hard to save a patient? Or are they more complaint-based? This will give you some insight into the team's organizational culture.

Reviewing case studies that highlight desired behaviors can also help drive changes to the organizational culture.

Adapting to a New Organizational Culture

Adapting to a new culture is both a requirement and a frequent occurrence as organizations grow and adapt to the global economy. When entering any new work environment, take time to assess the following:

- **The atmosphere:** Is the atmosphere tense? Calm? Chaotic? High energy? Low energy?
- **How people behave:** How do people interact with each other and with you? Are they formal or casual? Do they ask open-ended questions or closed-ended ones? Do they assume they already know the answers?
- **Team or individual focus:** Do employees use team language (we) or individual language (I)?
- **Flexibility and tradition:** Are traditions strictly maintained? Or do people focus more on innovation and change?
- **Level of planning:** Are employees willing to endure periods of disruption? Or do they adhere to strict arrangements during planning and implementation?
- **Values:** What do employees value in interactions, outcomes, and processes?

The Drive Home

Let's drive home the key points in this chapter:

- *Culture* refers to the characteristics historically shared by a group of people. This group may be self-determined or defined by outsiders looking in.
- Organizational culture and behaviors are defined by employees' life experiences, strengths, weaknesses, education, upbringing, and so forth.
- Cultural behavior is one small aspect of social traditions used in shaping group values and the cultural environment.
- Organizations can drive socialization by sharing stories, reviewing case studies that highlight desired behaviors, and having long-term members model the organizational values.
- Factors that drive organizational culture and behaviors include power and control, adaptation or deception, etiquette, formality, perception of time, hierarchy and gender, communication, and cliques and work ethics.
- Culture is an extension of the way people relate to one another.
- We must take the lead and model a strong and effective culture as it relates to social interactions, communication, shared interests and responsibilities, collaboration, and friendships.
- Informal leaders play key roles in ensuring that their organizational culture supports good relationships that empower everyone to do their work.
- We must show respect for the cultural and ethnic backgrounds of all families and colleagues.
- Your role in improving cultural behaviors includes understanding how organizations are dynamic and how your perception of the organization plays a key role in the enculturation, trust, and inspiration within it.

References

Barden, A. M., Quinn Griffin, M. T., Donahue, M., & Fitzpatrick, J. J. (2011). Shared governance and empowerment in registered nurses working in a hospital setting. *Nursing Administration Quarterly*, 35(3), 212–218. https://doi.org/10.1097/NAQ.0b013e3181ff3845

McKee, A. (2017). Happiness traps. *Harvard Business Review*. https://hbr.org/2017/09/happiness-traps

Pfeffer, J., & Veiga, J. F. (1999). Putting people first for organizational success. *Academy of Management Executive*, 13(2), 37–48. https://doi.org/10.5465/AME.1999.1899547

Traphagan, J. (2017, Jan. 6). We're thinking about organizational culture all wrong. *Harvard Business Review*. https://hbr.org/2017/01/were-thinking-about-organizational-culture-all-wrong

Watkins, M. D. (2013, May 15). What is organizational culture? And why should we care? *Harvard Business Review*. https://hbr.org/2013/05/what-is-organizational-culture

11
On Social Media

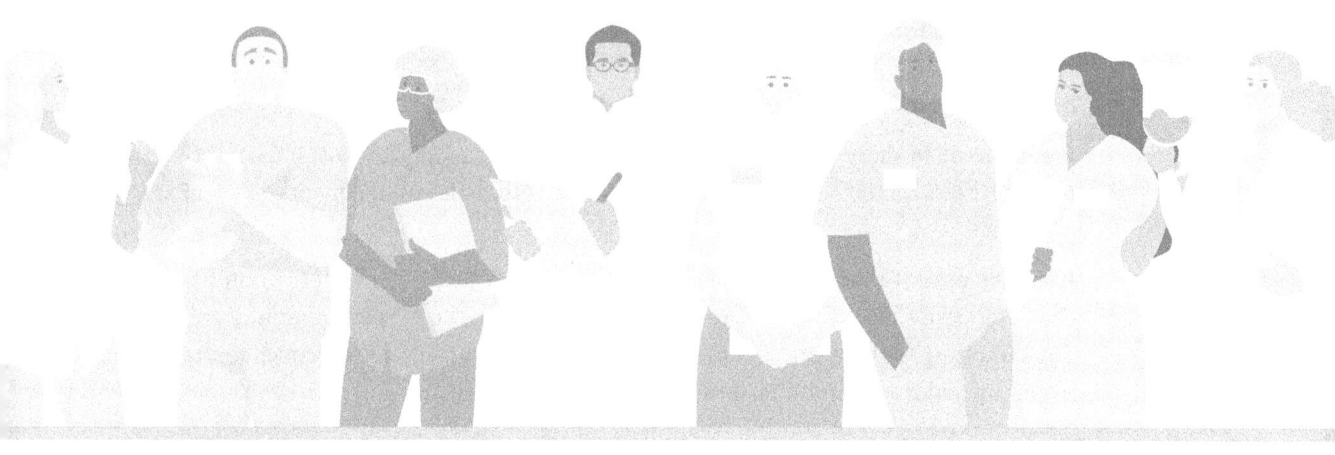

"You are what you share."
–Charles Leadbeater

Social media, also known as social networking, enables people to share personal and professional information using popular sites like Facebook, X (formerly Twitter), Instagram, Pinterest, LinkedIn, and more. We can quickly and easily share this information not only with our close circle of friends and colleagues but with anyone in the world.

Not surprisingly, nurses often use social media to communicate with, influence, and educate patients and the public at large. Yet, as with many things in life, there are pros and cons to using social media. As the use of social media continues to grow, so will the potential for both benefit and harm. In other words, while nurses should make the most of social media's positive aspects, they must also recognize its potential pitfalls.

The Pros of Social Media

Social media has brought about many benefits for society:

- **It's taught us a new language.** Tools like social media and texting have resulted in a completely new vocabulary. LOL (laugh out loud) and BTW (by the way) are just two of the hundreds of terms that are used in communications sent via social media or text.
- **It's reached a broader audience.** Before the internet, most people simply wrote letters or made phone calls to communicate with another person. Now we can reach hundreds or even thousands of people in seconds with just a single social media post.
- **It enables us to share more and more quickly.** People can quickly post important personal news on their Facebook page to share it with their entire network of friends all at once.
- **It's made us more succinct.** Certain social media sites, such as X, limit the number of characters you can use, which forces you to be more concise in your communication. The same goes for bloggers. Top bloggers know they have only a few seconds to draw a reader in, and they communicate accordingly!

Social Media for Healthcare Professionals: Networking and Staying Informed

Social media provides healthcare professionals an opportunity to connect and collaborate with peers around the world for personal and professional reasons. They join professional groups, participate in online forums, and engage in discussions with colleagues. This facilitates knowledge sharing, collaboration on research projects, and the exchange of best practices, ultimately enhancing the quality of care provided.

The top social media sites for healthcare professionals to access professional information, network, and stay updated are as follows:

- **LinkedIn:** A leading professional networking platform where healthcare professionals can connect with colleagues, join industry-specific groups, and access relevant news and articles shared by peers and thought leaders.
- **X (formerly Twitter):** A real-time information platform that allows healthcare professionals to follow medical journals, healthcare organizations, and influential individuals in the industry. It provides quick access to breaking news, research findings, and discussions on healthcare topics.
- **Doximity:** A professional network exclusively for healthcare professionals. It provides access to medical news, research articles, and collaboration tools to connect with colleagues and stay informed.
- **ResearchGate:** A platform for scientists and researchers, including healthcare professionals. It allows access to academic papers, collaboration opportunities, and the ability to connect with experts in specific fields.
- **Figure 1:** A social platform designed for healthcare professionals to share and discuss medical cases. It provides an opportunity to learn from real-life clinical scenarios and engage with a global community of healthcare professionals.
- **SERMO:** An online physician community that offers a platform for doctors to connect, collaborate, and share medical insights and experiences. It also provides access to medical news and research articles.
- **MedEdWorld:** An online community for healthcare educators. It provides access to educational resources, discussions on teaching methodologies, and opportunities for professional development.

Facebook for Nurses

Facebook offers many opportunities for nurses to join groups for work-related support, for organizing, and for peer-based support. This list is a small example of the nursing groups found on Facebook. While most of the groups listed here are public and you can view them when you are not logged into Facebook, a few require requests and cannot be viewed unless you are a Facebook member:

- **American Association of Legal Nurse Consultants:** The AALNC is dedicated to the professional enhancement and growth of RNs practicing in the specialty of legal nurse consulting.

- **Campaign for Statutory Minimum Nurse Patient Ratios:** This group supports a statutory minimum ratio of nurses to patients on hospital wards, with penalties for NHS trusts that fail to achieve those ratios.
- **Certified Emergency Nurses:** Although there are CENs throughout the world, the CEN exam is based on emergency nursing practice in the United States.
- **Nurse and Healthcare Worker Protection S.1788:** Senate Bill S.1788 would provide standards that would help mitigate potential injuries related to patient handling.
- **RNFA, Registered Nurse First Assistants:** This Facebook group page serves as a discussion area for RNFA interests.
- **Student Registered Nurse Anesthetist SRNA/CRNA Anesthesia Association:** This group is open to the nursing student, registered nurse, student registered nurse anesthetist (SRNA), certified registered nurse anesthetist (CRNA), and MD anesthesiologist.

Healthcare Professional X/Twitter Chats

Healthcare professionals participate in various X chats to engage in discussions, share insights, and exchange knowledge. While the popularity and frequency of specific X chats may vary over time, here are a few examples of popular healthcare-related X chats that professionals have used in the past:

- **#HCLDR:** Discusses healthcare leadership, innovation, patient-centered care, and improving the healthcare system.
- **#MedEd:** Explores topics related to medical education, including teaching methods, curriculum development, and technology in medical education.
- **#HealthXPh:** Focuses on the intersection of health and technology, exploring topics such as digital health, telemedicine, and health informatics.
- **#HITsm:** Covers the use of technology in healthcare, including electronic health records, interoperability, data privacy, and patient engagement.
- **#HPMChat:** Discusses issues related to palliative care, end-of-life care, pain management, and improving the quality of life for patients with serious illnesses.
- **#PrimaryCareChat:** Explores topics relevant to primary care providers, including preventive medicine, chronic disease management, and patient-centered primary care.
- **#RNChat:** Focuses on nursing-related topics, including professional development, nursing education, patient advocacy, and healthcare policy.

These are just a few examples, and there are many other healthcare-related X chats that professionals can participate in. It's a good idea to search for current and active X chats using relevant hashtags or keywords to find chats that align with your specific interests and expertise.

Information Resources on the Web for Healthcare Professionals

For professional healthcare resources, the following websites are widely regarded as valuable sources of information and tools for healthcare professionals, including research articles, clinical guidelines, drug information, and educational materials.

- **Agency for Healthcare Research and Quality** (AHRQ; www.ahrq.gov): Offers evidence-based research, quality improvement tools, and resources to support healthcare professionals in delivering effective and safe care.
- **American Medical Association** (AMA; www.ama-assn.org): Provides resources for physicians, including practice management tools, coding and billing information, advocacy resources, and professional development opportunities.
- **Centers for Disease Control and Prevention** (CDC; www.cdc.gov): An authoritative source for public health information. It provides guidelines, disease surveillance data, vaccine recommendations, and resources for healthcare professionals.
- **JAMA Network** (jamanetwork.com): Comprises a collection of highly regarded medical journals, such as *JAMA* (*Journal of the American Medical Association*), offering a wealth of research articles, clinical guidelines, and professional resources.
- *The Lancet* (www.thelancet.com): A renowned medical journal that publishes high-quality research articles, reviews, and commentary on various medical specialties.
- **MedPage Today** (www.medpagetoday.com): A trusted source of medical news and education for healthcare professionals. It offers daily updates on clinical research, medical breakthroughs, and expert opinions.
- **Medscape** (www.medscape.com): Provides a wide range of resources for healthcare professionals, including medical news, clinical reference tools, drug information, expert commentary, and continuing medical education opportunities.
- **National Institutes of Health** (NIH; www.nih.gov): Provides information on cutting-edge research, clinical trials, grants, and funding opportunities. It also offers resources for healthcare professionals, including medical literature and educational materials.

- **PubMed** (pubmed.ncbi.nlm.nih.gov): A database of biomedical literature provided by the National Library of Medicine. It allows healthcare professionals to access millions of research articles, clinical studies, and medical journals.
- **UpToDate** (www.uptodate.com): An evidence-based clinical decision support resource that offers in-depth articles, drug information, patient education materials, and expert recommendations on various medical topics.
- **World Health Organization** (WHO; www.who.int): Offers global health data, guidelines, publications, and reports on various health topics. It serves as a valuable resource for healthcare professionals working in international health.

Please note that the websites mentioned above are provided as examples and may not cover all the specific content mentioned. It's always important to visit reputable sources for accurate and up-to-date information.

Healthcare Research Best Practices

Healthcare professionals should exercise caution and critically evaluate the information they come across on social media platforms, ensuring it comes from reputable sources and aligns with evidence-based practices. When looking up healthcare information professionally, it's important to follow a systematic approach to ensure the information you find is reliable, accurate, and up to date. Here are some steps to consider:

1. **Start with trusted sources.** Begin your search by consulting reputable and authoritative sources of healthcare information. These may include government health agencies, professional healthcare organizations, academic institutions, and peer-reviewed journals. Examples of reliable sources include the CDC, WHO, NIH, and respected medical journals like the *New England Journal of Medicine* or *JAMA*.

2. **Use dedicated healthcare databases.** Utilize specialized healthcare databases to access high-quality research literature, clinical guidelines, and evidence-based practice resources. Examples of widely used healthcare databases include PubMed, Embase, Cochrane Library, and CINAHL. These databases provide access to a wealth of peer-reviewed articles and other healthcare-related content.

3. **Employ advanced search techniques.** When searching for healthcare information, use advanced search techniques to refine your results. This may involve combining relevant keywords, using Boolean operators (AND, OR, NOT), specifying search filters (e.g., publication date, study type), and utilizing subject headings or MeSH terms (in PubMed) to enhance the accuracy and relevance of your search.

4. **Evaluate sources and information.** Assess the credibility and reliability of the sources and information you find. Consider factors such as the expertise and reputation of the authors or organizations, the presence of proper citations and references, the currency of the information, and whether the content aligns with current scientific knowledge. Be cautious of sources that lack transparency, have bias, or make unsupported claims.

5. **Cross-reference information.** Verify information by cross-referencing multiple sources. If you encounter conflicting information or something seems questionable, consult additional reputable sources to gain a well-rounded understanding of the topic. Look for consensus among trusted sources to ensure the information is reliable.

6. **Stay updated.** Healthcare information evolves rapidly, so it's crucial to stay updated with the latest research, guidelines, and advancements in your field. Subscribe to reputable healthcare journals or newsletters, follow trusted professional organizations and experts on social media, and attend conferences or webinars to stay abreast of current knowledge.

7. **Consult colleagues and experts.** Engage in discussions with colleagues, mentors, or subject matter experts within your professional network. Collaborating and exchanging information with knowledgeable peers can provide valuable insights and help validate your findings.

Remember, healthcare information should always be interpreted in the appropriate context and should not replace professional expertise or clinical judgment. When in doubt, consult with healthcare professionals or specialists for personalized advice and guidance.

Social Media as a Powerful Tool for Health Education and Promotion

Healthcare professionals, including nurses, use social media as a powerful tool for health promotion. Here are some ways they utilize social media platforms for this purpose:

- **Health education:** Healthcare professionals share accurate and reliable health information on social media platforms to educate the public. They create and share posts, videos, infographics, and articles on various health topics, including disease prevention, healthy lifestyle choices, and symptom recognition. By providing accessible and understandable information, they empower individuals to make informed decisions about their health.

- **Public health campaigns:** Social media offers healthcare professionals an effective way to launch and promote public health campaigns. They create dedicated hashtags, develop compelling content, and engage with the online community to raise awareness about specific health issues or initiatives. This helps in disseminating important health messages to a wide audience, encouraging behavior change, and promoting positive health outcomes.
- **Community engagement:** Social media platforms allow healthcare professionals to engage directly with communities and individuals. They participate in discussions, answer questions, and provide guidance on health-related concerns. By actively engaging with their audience, healthcare professionals foster a sense of trust and promote dialogue around important health topics.
- **Patient support and empowerment:** Healthcare professionals use social media to provide support and empower patients. They create online communities, support groups, or patient advocacy networks where individuals can connect, share experiences, and find emotional support. These platforms serve as a valuable resource for patients to access information, seek advice, and connect with others facing similar health challenges.
- **Advocacy and policy influence:** Social media empowers healthcare professionals to advocate for healthcare policy changes and raise awareness about healthcare disparities. They utilize their platforms to share personal stories, research findings, and evidence-based information to support their advocacy efforts. By mobilizing their online networks, healthcare professionals can drive public support and influence policymakers to make positive changes in healthcare.
- **Influencing positive health behaviors:** Healthcare professionals leverage social media's reach and influence to promote positive health behaviors. They share success stories, practical tips, and motivational content to encourage individuals to adopt healthy lifestyles, engage in physical activity, practice self-care, and follow evidence-based guidelines for disease prevention and management.
- **Disseminating research and evidence:** Social media provides healthcare professionals with a platform to share research findings, studies, and evidence-based guidelines with a broader audience. They can summarize complex research in an accessible format, increasing the visibility and impact of important scientific discoveries. This

> "There is something uniquely pleasing about being involved in social media. For me personally it helps to justify that I am on the right path in life. Now many may argue that you should rely on yourself for personal fulfillment, but humans seek the social interaction of others. We take comfort in knowing we aren't alone in this world and that there are others like us who share the same opinions that we do."
>
> –Brittney Wilson, 2012, para. 12

helps bridge the gap between research and practice, ensuring that the latest evidence informs healthcare decisions.

By leveraging the power of social media, healthcare professionals can reach a vast audience, promote health literacy, and inspire positive health behaviors. It allows for real-time communication, engagement, and collaboration, extending the impact of their work beyond traditional healthcare settings.

Examples of Effective Health Promotion in Social Media

Here are some specific examples of how healthcare professionals have used social media for health promotion, along with corresponding websites:

- **The American Heart Association's #CheckIt Challenge website: https://www.heart.org**

  The American Heart Association launched the #CheckIt Challenge, an online campaign aimed at raising awareness about high blood pressure and encouraging individuals to monitor their blood pressure regularly. They utilized social media platforms, including Twitter (now X) and Instagram, to share informative posts, videos, and testimonials from individuals sharing their blood pressure measurements. The campaign encouraged participants to get their blood pressure checked, share their results using the hashtag #CheckIt, and nominate others to participate.

- **Mayo Clinic's Facebook Live Sessions website: https://www.mayoclinic.org**

  Mayo Clinic, a renowned healthcare organization, conducts regular Facebook Live sessions on various health topics. These sessions feature expert healthcare professionals discussing specific conditions, treatments, or general health advice. Viewers can engage in real time by asking questions, which are addressed by the experts during the livestream. The Facebook Live sessions provide an interactive platform for healthcare professionals to educate and engage with the audience in an accessible format.

- **World Health Organization's (WHO) X Updates website: https://www.who.int**

  The WHO utilizes its X account (@WHO) to provide timely updates on global health issues, outbreaks, and public health emergencies. They share important information about disease prevention, vaccination campaigns, and health guidelines. Through their X presence, WHO reaches millions of followers, sharing accurate and up-to-date health information to promote public health awareness and address misinformation.

- **Nursing organizations' online communities websites:**
    - The American Nurses Association (ANA): https://www.nursingworld.org
    - The Royal College of Nursing (RCN): https://www.rcn.org.uk

    Nursing organizations, such as the ANA and RCN, host online communities and forums where nurses can connect, share experiences, and access resources. These platforms provide opportunities for networking, mentorship, and professional development. Nurses can engage in discussions, seek advice, and share best practices, fostering a supportive and collaborative environment within the nursing community.

- **Dr. Mike's YouTube Channel: https://www.youtube.com/doctor.mike**

    Dr. Mikhail Varshavski, known as "Dr. Mike," is a physician and social media influencer who uses his YouTube channel to share health tips, medical advice, and educational content. He covers a wide range of health topics, debunking myths and providing evidence-based information in an engaging and accessible manner. Dr. Mike's channel has garnered a large following, allowing him to reach a broad audience with his health promotion messages.

The Cons of Social Media

Just as there are many advantages to using social media, there are also some disadvantages:

- **Distractions and disruptions:** It has become more and more difficult to hold a conversation, meeting, or conference without people checking their smartphones.
- **No body language or tonal cues:** Another drawback is that you can't read the other person's tone or body language. (This is why I often end my posts, texts, and emails with a smiley face or a winking face—so the reader or recipient knows my true intentions.)
- **Inappropriate or inaccurate content:** Unfortunately, the posting of inappropriate and/or inaccurate content is widespread.
- **Algorithmic bias:** Social media algorithms may unintentionally favor certain content, perspectives, or groups over others. This can result in a skewed presentation of information, reinforcing existing biases and limiting exposure to diverse viewpoints.
- **Filter bubbles:** Users often engage with content that aligns with their existing beliefs and preferences. This can create filter bubbles, where individuals are exposed to a narrow range of perspectives, leading to reinforcement of their existing biases and limited exposure to alternative viewpoints.
- **Selective exposure:** Users have the ability to curate their online experience by choosing who to follow and what content to engage with. This selective exposure can lead to a distorted view of reality, as users may avoid information that challenges their beliefs.

- **Spread of misinformation:** Social media can be a breeding ground for the rapid spread of misinformation and fake news. Biases in content creation and sharing can contribute to the dissemination of false or misleading information, potentially influencing public opinion.
- **Targeted advertising and profiling:** Social media platforms often use targeted advertising based on user data. This can lead to the reinforcement of stereotypes and the creation of profiles that may not accurately represent individuals, contributing to biased targeting.
- **Online harassment and hate speech:** Biases can manifest in the form of online harassment and hate speech. Certain groups may be disproportionately targeted, leading to a negative and harmful online environment.
- **Manipulation of public opinion:** The ability to manipulate content visibility and engagement on social media can be exploited to influence public opinion. This can have political and social consequences, with biased information shaping people's perceptions.

Social Media for Healthcare Professionals: Navigating Ethical and Legal Issues

Nurses who post inappropriate content on social media are at a high risk of violating state and federal laws. These laws were initiated to protect patient privacy and confidentiality. Misuse of social media may have significant consequences, including civil and criminal liabilities. Nurses may also face personal liability, which means they may be individually sued for defamation, invasion of privacy, or harassment.

Often the arbiter in cases involving the misuse of social media is the state board of nursing (BON). The laws that chart the basis for punitive action by a state BON can vary between jurisdictions. According to the National Council of State Boards of Nursing (NCSBN, 2011b), a state BON may investigate reports of inappropriate postings on social media on any of the following grounds:

- Unprofessional or unethical conduct
- Maladministration of patient records
- Revealing a privileged communication
- Breach of confidentiality

Some inappropriate postings are considered patient abuse, a Health Insurance Portability and Accountability Act (HIPAA) violation, or exploitation. The NCSBN explains:

> HIPAA regulations are intended to protect patient privacy and confidentiality by defining individually identifiable information and establishing how this information may be used, by whom and under what circumstances. The definition of individually identifiable information includes any information that relates to the past, present or future physical or mental health of an individual, or provides enough information that leads someone to believe the information could be used to identify an individual. (NCSBN, 2018, p. 7)

If a nurse is found guilty of inappropriate conduct, the BON may impose a fine or confiscate the nurse's license.

The Consequences of Violating Patient Privacy

A 2010 survey of boards of nursing (BON) conducted by the NCSBN indicated that an overwhelming majority of responding BONs (33 of the 46 respondents) reported receiving complaints about nurses who had violated patient privacy by posting photos or information about patients on social networking sites. The majority of BONs who had received such a complaint (26 of the 33) reported taking disciplinary actions based on these complaints. Actions taken by these BONs ranged from censuring the nurse to issuing a letter of concern to placing conditions on the nurse's license to suspending the nurse's license (NCSBN, 2011b).

It is also crucial for healthcare professionals to familiarize themselves with their organization's policies, professional codes of conduct, and regulatory guidelines specific to social media use, which may be more limiting than state or federal laws.

Doing Your Due Diligence

Nurses need to be mindful of their ethical and legal obligations to patients and the professional boundaries that are warranted whenever social media is used. It is a nurse's due diligence to be aware of and adhere to legal, regulatory, institutional, and/or employer guidelines and policies. Familiarize yourself with your employer's social media policies and guidelines. Many healthcare organizations have specific rules regarding social media use, which may include restrictions on discussing work-related matters, posting photos from the workplace, or representing the organization without proper authorization.

Using Social Media for Good

Brittney Wilson, also known as the Nerdy Nurse, is an award-winning author and national speaker on social media issues, bullying, and informatics. She argues that nurses can use social media as a way of gaining confidence and feeling empowered through conversations about issues and solutions, increasing knowledge, and even blogging "to document your personal experiences and connect to others who have experienced the same" (Wilson, 2012, para. 6). She explains, "Social media, and in particular blogging, have given me a connection to the world that I would never have otherwise. I am able to meet and become friends with people based purely upon our common interests without any dependence on our relative geographies" (Wilson, 2012, para. 13).

The following recommendations—both do's and don'ts—provide guidance for the appropriate use of social media (ANA, 2011; McGinnis, 2011; NCSBN, 2011a, 2011b, 2018; Spector & Kappel, 2012).

Social Media Do's for Healthcare Professionals

- **Engage responsibly:** Engage in respectful and meaningful discussions on social media platforms. Be mindful of your words and maintain a positive and empathetic attitude. Strive to uplift the profession.

- **Educate, don't diagnose:** When sharing healthcare information or advice, be clear that you are not providing medical diagnoses or treatment recommendations. Encourage individuals to consult with healthcare professionals for personalized guidance. Share evidence-based information from reputable sources to promote health literacy.

- **Monitor privacy settings:** Regularly review and update your privacy settings on social media platforms. Ensure that your personal information is protected and that only approved connections have access to your content. Be cautious when accepting friend requests or connections from individuals you do not know personally.

- **Stay informed about social media trends:** Social media platforms and their policies are constantly evolving. Stay informed about changes in privacy settings, guidelines, and best practices. Regularly review your own social media presence to ensure compliance with current standards.

- **Protect patient privacy and confidentiality:** Protecting patient privacy is paramount. Healthcare professionals should never disclose any identifiable patient information, including names, images, or specific case details, without obtaining proper consent. It is crucial to comply with legal and regulatory requirements, such as HIPAA in the United States, which governs the privacy and security of patient health information.

- **Maintain professionalism and integrity:** Healthcare professionals should maintain professionalism and integrity when using social media. This involves refraining from engaging in unprofessional behavior, such as making derogatory or offensive remarks about patients, colleagues, or healthcare institutions. Professionals should remember that their online presence reflects their professional image and can impact their reputation.
- **Separate personal and professional profiles:** It is advisable for healthcare professionals to have separate personal and professional social media profiles. This helps distinguish between personal opinions and professional recommendations or information shared. Maintaining separate profiles also reduces the risk of inadvertently mixing personal and professional content.
- **Practice with transparency and disclosure:** When sharing professional information on social media, healthcare professionals should be transparent about their professional identity, qualifications, and any potential conflicts of interest. Disclosing potential conflicts of interest ensures transparency and helps audiences evaluate the information in an informed manner.
- **Provide accurate and evidence-based information:** Healthcare professionals have a responsibility to ensure the accuracy and reliability of the information they share on social media. It is essential to rely on evidence-based sources and reputable research. Sharing false or misleading information can have serious consequences for patients and the public and can undermine trust in the profession.
- **Respect colleagues and professional boundaries:** Healthcare professionals should demonstrate respect for their colleagues on social media. This involves refraining from sharing confidential or sensitive information about other healthcare professionals or institutions. Maintaining professional boundaries on social media is crucial to preserving trust and fostering a positive professional environment.
- **Maintain professional relationships with patients:** Healthcare professionals should be cautious when engaging with patients on social media. It is important to maintain appropriate professional boundaries and avoid engaging in therapeutic or personal relationships with patients outside of established professional settings. Social media should not be used as a substitute for formal medical advice or treatment.
- **Practice informed consent:** Before sharing patient stories, images, or testimonials on social media, healthcare professionals must obtain informed consent from the patients involved. This ensures that patients understand the implications of sharing their information and have the opportunity to make an informed decision regarding their privacy.

- **Be mindful of your digital footprint:** Healthcare professionals should be mindful of their digital footprint on social media platforms. It is essential to regularly review and manage online presence, ensuring that the content aligns with professional and ethical standards. Healthcare professionals should consider the potential long-term impact of their online activity on their professional reputation and act accordingly.

- **Handle negative feedback professionally:** If you receive negative feedback or criticism on social media, respond in a professional and constructive manner. Avoid engaging in arguments or becoming defensive. Instead, take the opportunity to provide clarification, apologize if necessary, and address concerns offline or through appropriate channels.

- **Realize nothing is truly anonymous online:** Be cognizant that everything you post online is public and can be copied and redistributed (regardless of your privacy settings).

- **Report online trolling or abuse:** Report inappropriate material and take action if you are the subject of complaints or abuse on social media.

- **Be aware that you may be communicating via social media even when you think you aren't:** For example, if you fail to accept someone's friend request or you ignore something someone posts on your Facebook page or X feed, that person may take that to mean you don't like them or care about them—even if it was just an innocent oversight.

Social Media Don'ts for Healthcare Professionals

- **Post patient information:** It is strictly prohibited to share any identifiable patient information, including names, images, medical histories, or any other personally identifiable information. Respecting patient confidentiality and privacy is paramount. Photographs or videos of patients or distribution of any electronic media of any patient-related information—except for professional reasons—is a violation of patient confidentiality and privacy. Such electronic images and recordings should only be used on private and encrypted media and with written consent granted.

- **Reveal sensitive or confidential information:** Healthcare professionals should avoid posting any sensitive or confidential information related to their workplace, colleagues, or healthcare institutions. This includes discussions about specific cases, internal processes, or any information that could compromise the security or reputation of individuals or organizations.

- **Identify your employer on your social media profiles:** While you may choose to identify your profession in either personal or professional profiles, it's best not to include the specific name of your employer.

- **Post derogatory or offensive content:** Healthcare professionals should not engage in posting or sharing content that is derogatory, offensive, or discriminatory towards patients, colleagues, their employer, or any other individuals or groups. Upholding professionalism, fostering a positive work environment, and showing respect for all individuals are essential.

- **Share unverified or misleading information:** Healthcare professionals should not share unverified or misleading information on social media. It is crucial to ensure that any information or content shared is evidence-based, accurate, and from reputable sources. Misinformation can have serious consequences for patients and the public.

- **Pose personal opinions as professional advice:** Healthcare professionals should not present personal opinions or anecdotes as professional advice on social media. It is important to distinguish between personal opinions and evidence-based recommendations. Sharing professional knowledge and expertise should be done responsibly and based on accepted standards of practice.

- **Commit any violation of professional codes and regulations:** Healthcare professionals should avoid posting content that violates the professional codes and regulations of their respective disciplines. This includes adhering to ethical guidelines, legal obligations, and the policies set forth by their professional associations and regulatory bodies.

- **Disclose confidential workplace information:** Posting confidential workplace information, such as internal policies, procedures, or proprietary information, is strictly prohibited. Maintaining the trust and integrity of the healthcare institution is essential.

- **Promote personal or commercial interests:** Healthcare professionals should avoid using social media solely for the promotion of personal or commercial interests. Balancing professional integrity with appropriate engagement and educational content is key.

- **Participate in inappropriate or unprofessional behavior:** Any content that exhibits inappropriate or unprofessional behavior, such as engaging in online disputes, cyberbullying, or violating social media platform rules, should be avoided. Healthcare professionals should uphold professional standards and contribute positively to the online community.

- **Accept patients as social network "friends":** It is not advised to accept patients as friends on personal social media accounts. This helps to maintain patient confidentiality, uphold professional boundaries, prevent misinterpretation, avoid favoritism, protect personal privacy, adhere to workplace policies, and consider legal and ethical considerations.

Remember, your actions on social media can have a lasting impact on your professional reputation and the trust patients place in you as a healthcare provider. By following these guidelines, you can use social media as a tool for professional development, knowledge sharing, and positive engagement while upholding ethical standards.

References

American Nurses Association. (2011). *ANA's principles for social networking and the nurse.* https://www.nursingworld.org/~4af4f2/globalassets/docs/ana/ethics/social-networking.pdf

McGinnis, M. S. (2011). Using Facebook as your professional social media presence. *Imprint, 58*(4), 36–39.

National Council of State Boards of Nursing. (2011a). *ANA and NCSBN unite to provide guidelines on social media and networking for nurses.* https://www.globenewswire.com/news-release/2011/10/19/1121644/0/en/ANA-and-NCSBN-Unite-to-Provide-Guidelines-on-Social-Media-and-Networking-for-Nurses.html

National Council of State Boards of Nursing. (2011b). *White paper: A nurse's guide to the use of social media.* https://www.ncsbn.org/public-files/Social_Media.pdf

National Council of State Boards of Nursing. (2018). *A nurse's guide to the use of social media.* https://www.ncsbn.org/public-files/NCSBN_SocialMedia.pdf

Spector, N., & Kappel, D. (2012). Guidelines for using electronic and social media: The regulatory perspective. *The Online Journal of Issues in Nursing, 17*(3). https://doi.org/10.3912/OJIN.Vol17No03Man01

Wilson, B. (2012, June 6). *Six reasons why nurses should use social media.* The Nerdy Nurse. https://thenerdynurse.com/6-reasons-why-nurses-should-use-social-media/

12
Conclusion

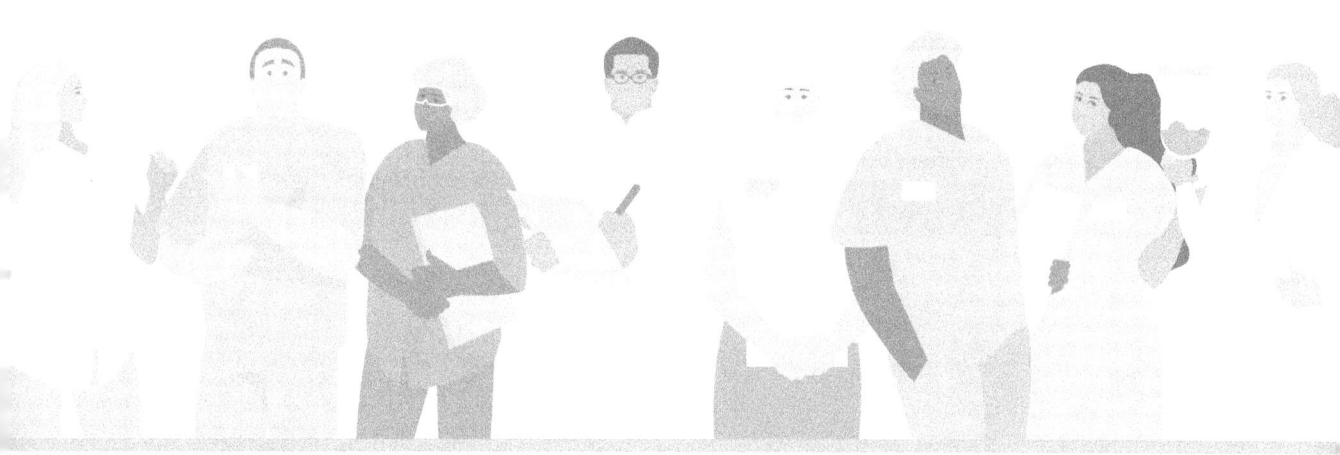

Transparency and clear communication are critical to creating a culture of safety in healthcare. Patients, nurses, nurse leaders and other leaders, and providers must consistently practice clear, empathic, two-way communication that is respectful to the beliefs of others. Effective communication is key to providing safe, high-quality care.

Effective communication within a healthcare organization results in two benefits:

- Patients become more informed and more involved in decision-making. Effective communication creates an environment in which patients are comfortable asking questions, sharing their perceptions, and owning their healthcare.
- Employees at all levels in the organization become more proactive in solving problems and resolving conflict quickly and respectfully. They also feel they have a worthwhile role in the organization. In other words, regardless of title, employees feel their roles and responsibilities are essential to the organization's mission and vision.

More than that, effective communication connects people—the antidote to practically any toxic situation. Without effective communication, misinterpretations and assumptions are more likely, which leads to poor outcomes for everyone.

Strategies to stimulate effective interprofessional communication include the following:

- Service-recovery readiness
- Purposeful patient hourly rounding
- Bedside shift reporting
- Conducting post-discharge phone calls
- Using open-ended questions
- Implementing scripts to ensure key talking points are conveyed
- Actively listening
- Using teach-back methods to ensure patients have the knowledge, skill, and ability to act on new information
- Implementing purposeful leader-staff rounding

Of course, none of these strategies are helpful if there isn't authenticity behind the words!

On the subject of scripting: You need not memorize these scripts. In fact, it might be better if you don't. Otherwise, you might sound, well, scripted. Instead, think of scripting as a framework, with handy acronyms to guide your conversations.

Also, regardless of what message you need to convey, your body language must match your words. To ensure this, the BEST approach must be hardwired. This approach will help you remember to use acronyms such as HEARD or SBAR to recall key talking points, to remain cognizant of your body language, to tap into your emotional intelligence and competence, and to use various scripting techniques within the acronym. For example, use 3WITH to remind yourself to ask open-ended questions.

Implementing effective interprofessional and patient communication is simply the right thing to do, and doing the right thing has its benefits. One of these is keeping your job. I am not talking about avoiding any punitive measures that may come if you fail to communicate well. I mean that effective communication can help ensure the fiscal stability of your organization. Recall that HCAHPS scores, which measure patient experience, are one of the measures used by the Centers for Medicare & Medicaid Services (CMS) to calculate reimbursement payments to hospitals. Higher scores mean higher rates of reimbursement. Higher scores, which are published online, also increase the likelihood that potential patients will choose your facility over another.

So, what does all this have to do with effective communication? Simple. Several core questions in the HCAHPS pertain to communication. Indeed, many studies have found evidence of a correlation among communication, patient experience, and HCAHPS scores:

- Jun et al. (2020) found that the improvement of HCAHPS scores is linked to nurse-led interventions, particularly nursing rounds. These rounds have shown positive effects on various outcomes, such as increased HCAHPS scores, reduced falls, and decreased patients' call light use. However, a systematic review noted inconsistencies in the implementation, performance, measurement, and analysis of nursing rounds, with weak evidence for definitive conclusions. Despite this, nursing rounds remain an area where nurses can enhance patients' experiences.

- This study also determined that the transition from hospitals to home is considered vulnerable. The stress of this transition for patients often overrides discharge education and instruction. In the context of HCAHPS, discharge education and follow-up phone calls within 48 hours post-discharge have gained attention as areas for improvement in patient satisfaction.

- According to research conducted by Press Ganey Associates of more than 3,000 hospitals, scores in the Nurse-Patient Communication domain in HCAHPS affected ratings in the Responsiveness of Hospital Staff, Pain Management, Communication About Medication, and Overall Rating domains (Press Ganey, 2013). In other words, when scores in the Nurse-Patient Communication domain rise, so do the scores in these other domains (and vice versa), which can have a profound effect on the overall survey score.

Effective communication serves as a foundational element in engaging the workforce. Research demonstrates that robust communication among healthcare team members plays a crucial role in shaping the quality of working relationships and job satisfaction (Agency for Healthcare Research and Quality, 2023). Specifically, clear communication regarding task allocation and responsibilities has been linked to a decrease in workforce turnover, particularly within nursing staff.

Collectively, these findings suggest that when healthcare professionals communicate adeptly—conveying crucial information in a timely and easily comprehensible manner, explicitly outlining orders or instructions, and addressing questions thoroughly—they contribute to safer, higher-quality care. Moreover, studies indicate that such care is not only more cost-efficient but also more cost-effective, essential considerations in the context of value-based healthcare.

In contrast, inadequate communication among care team members and with patients, family members, and post-acute care facilities during discharge can result in confusion regarding follow-up care and medications. This confusion may lead to unnecessary readmissions and potential malpractice litigation. In a comprehensive study utilizing six years of data from nearly 3,000 acute-care hospitals, researchers found that communication between caregivers and patients has the most significant impact on reducing readmissions. Specifically, prioritizing patient communication, in addition to complying with evidence-based care standards, could, on average, reduce a hospital's readmission rate by 5% (Senot et al., 2015).

The recognition that communication influences the safety, quality, and experience of care, as well as caregiver engagement, aligns with research linking these critical performance areas to patient-centered care. It also corresponds with cross-domain analyses indicating the high interrelation of these elements with each other and with financial outcomes (Press Ganey, 2017).

Given that communication is the common thread tying these areas together, health systems aiming to improve safety, quality, and patient-centeredness must identify and eliminate barriers to effective communication. They should adopt strategies that enhance caregivers' professional and interpersonal communication skills.

To achieve this goal, several evidence-based best practices can enhance communication skills and improve outcomes, such as implementing a comprehensive provider/team communication strategy, investing in communication skills training for all staff, and making leadership support for communication initiatives highly visible. Leadership must create an open communication environment by modeling appropriate behavior, setting expectations, and investing in support systems within the organization's structure. Leaders and managers at all levels should promote patient-centered communication as a requirement for providing safe, high-quality care.

The ability to explain, listen, and empathize significantly impacts relationships with patients and colleagues, influencing individual and organizational performance in clinical quality, the experience of care, and financial outcomes. Therefore, health systems should invest in monitoring and developing these skills in the current workforce, while the industry as a whole should support initiatives focused on building these skills in the physicians, nurses, and healthcare workers of the future.

In summary, elevating communication to facilitate the transformation from a volume-based to a value-based healthcare system is a critical imperative. While numerous barriers, be they structural, procedural, or cultural, stand in our way, a concerted effort in research, education, and sustained support is key to surmounting these challenges. This journey toward success mandates the establishment of clear objectives, the identification of champions, the cultivation of consensus, and an adaptive approach informed by experience.

Central to this transformation is the embrace of effective communication encompassing both verbal and nonverbal elements. Consistent practice of clear, empathic, two-way communication, underscored by emotional intelligence and cultural competence, is a shared responsibility. Moreover, the power of social media in enhancing communication cannot be overlooked. Utilizing platforms such as social media can amplify our reach, engage diverse audiences, and foster collaborative dialogues on healthcare.

As healthcare professionals, we are entrusted with the responsibility to champion effective communication across various channels, including social media, all while embodying emotional intelligence. This comprehensive approach not only enhances patient care within our immediate scope but also contributes to the broader narrative of transforming healthcare into a value-driven, patient-centric paradigm.

References

Agency for Healthcare Research and Quality. (2023). *TeamSTEPPS: Strategies and tools to enhance performance and patient safety*. https://psnet.ahrq.gov/issue/teamstepps-strategies-and-tools-enhance-performance-and-patient-safety

Jun, J., Stern, K., & Djukic, M. (2020). Integrative review of the interventions for improving patients' experiences revealed in quality improvement projects. *Journal of Patient Experience, 7*(6), 882–892. https://doi.org/10.1177/2374373520925271

Press Ganey. (2013). *The rising tide measure: Communication with nurses*. https://www.semanticscholar.org/paper/The-Rising-Tide-Measure-%3A-Communication-With-Nurses/594d6268ae537be86b4dfc6153ffc9adf0cf3289

Press Ganey. (2017). *Achieving excellence: The convergence of safety, quality, experience and caregiver engagement*. https://health.pressganey.com/hubfs/Achieving-Excellence-The-Convergence-of-Safety-Quality-Experience-and-Caregiver-Engagement.pdf

Senot, C., Chandrasekaran, A., Ward, P. T., Tucker, A. L., & Moffatt-Bruce, S. D. (2015, July 21). The impact of combining conformance and experiential quality on hospitals' readmissions and cost performance. *Management Science, 62*(3), 829–848. https://doi.org/10.1287/mnsc.2014.2141

A

Sample Rounding Template

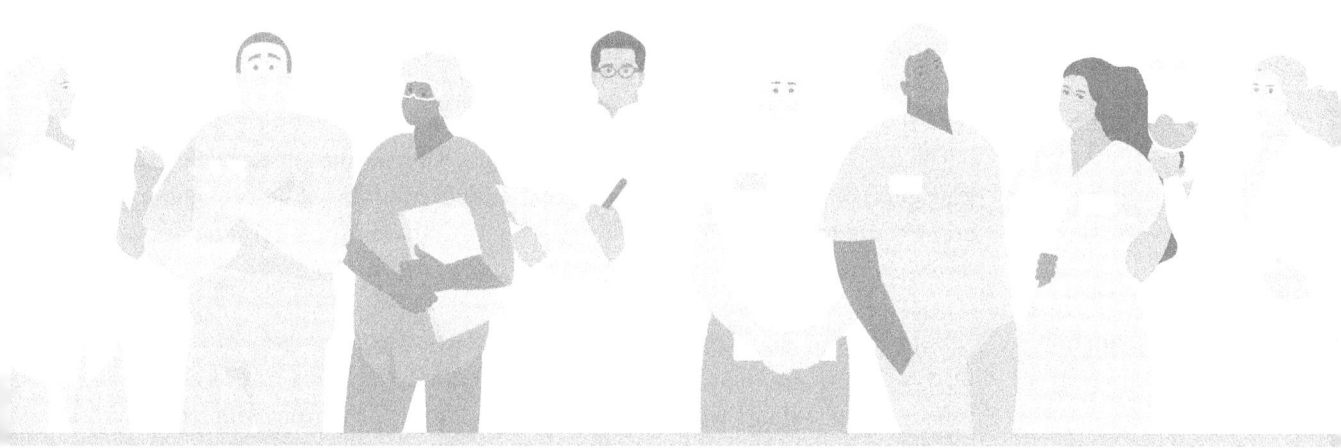

Sample Transformational Rounding Template

The purpose of this template is to provide you with a comprehensive tool for rounding with staff or other direct reports. If you have fewer than 30 direct reports, it is advised you meet monthly. Bimonthly or even quarterly rounding is recommended if you have more than 30 direct reports.

Sample Transformational Rounding Template

Leader name:_____Date: _____

Direct report name:_____Department:_____

Sample Impromptu Scripting for AIDET (Role Model; Studer, 2004)

Acknowledge	"I appreciate the time you are taking out of your busy schedule to meet with me."
Introduce	"As you may know, my role in the organization is to help promote a healthy workplace environment." (Introduce your name and role if this is the first meeting.)
Duration	"Our one on one will take approximately 15 minutes to one hour, depending on the detail of our responses. Every month, I will ask you approximately nine questions that will help me gain a better understanding of how things are going and will also give you the opportunity to share any concerns or feedback with me."
Explanation	"The purpose of our meetings is to provide shared transparency. We will discuss career planning, rewards, and recognition, as well as how we can improve current systems and processes. Please feel free to be upfront with me. Your opinion matters."
Thank you	"Thank you for taking time to talk with me. Your feedback is appreciated."

Individual Trust and Succession Planning

1. "Tell me what you feel is working well. This can include initiatives on our unit, within the organization, or even at home." (Make personal connection.)

    Notes:

    _____
    _____
    _____

    a. If positive, notes are made to follow up in future meetings.

    b. If negative, ask what solutions the employee may have to help the situation. Notes are made to follow up in the next meeting. If personal, offer Employee Assistance Program information (if applicable).

2. Tell me about where you would like to see your career in one year. Five years? Ten years? (This question doesn't have to be asked at every meeting but should be incorporated in question 2 as a talking point and, depending on the answer, questions 2a through 2d can be interwoven in the conversation.)

    Notes:

    _____
    _____
    _____

    a. "Based on your career goal, have you taken any steps (e.g., reading, education, committees, etc.) to achieve this goal?"

    _____
    _____

    b. "Is there anything pertinent you have heard or learned that you would like to share at the next staff meeting?" (This question is great to incorporate if the nurse is in school or has recently attended a conference, etc.)

    _____
    _____

c. "Have you implemented any actions to achieve your career goal?"

_____
_____

d. "Is there anything I can do now to help you achieve your short-term/long-term goals?"

_____
_____

Healthy Workplace Environment

1. "Are there any systems or processes that do not meet your expectations?" (Circle) "In other words, have you ever asked yourself why something is so complex when you feel it could have been done so much easier?"

    a. No—all systems and processes meet my expectations.

    b. Yes—please provide solutions on how to meet your expectations.

    _____
    _____

2. "Are there any systems or processes that exceed your expectations?" (Circle.) "In other words, what have you seen or done in our unit or organization that made you say, 'Wow! That was great!'"

    a. No—all systems and processes meet my expectations.

    b. Yes—please provide your rationale for why this exceeds your expectations.

    _____
    _____

Rewards and Recognition

1. "Do you feel any of your coworkers have gone 'above and beyond' their role?"

   Name _____

   Situation (Describe the event.)

   _____
   _____
   _____

   Action (What specifically did the coworker do?)

   _____
   _____
   _____

   Response (What was the specific outcome?)

   _____
   _____
   _____

2. "Do you feel any providers (physicians or mid-level providers) have gone 'above and beyond' their role?"

   Name _____

   Situation (Describe the event.)

   _____
   _____
   _____

Action (What specifically did the provider do?)

_____
_____
_____

Response (What was the specific outcome?)

_____
_____
_____

3. "Do you feel any other departments have gone 'above and beyond' their role?"

Name _____

Situation (Describe the event.)

_____
_____
_____

Action (What specifically did the department do?)

_____
_____
_____

Response (What was the specific outcome?)

_____
_____
_____

Coaching

1. "We all experience difficult situations at different times. Have you experienced any since our last meeting?" (Circle one)

    a. No issues at this time to be addressed.

    b. Yes—please provide details about the situation.

    Situation

    _____
    _____

    Action

    _____
    _____

    Response

    _____
    _____

    c. Use the TELL acronym to address tough issues or difficult conversations that you need to address.

    Time and place to talk.

    _____
    _____

    Explain and explore perspectives.

    _____
    _____

Listen with empathy.

_____
_____

Learn.

_____
_____

Thank you.

"Thank you for meeting with me. Is there anything I can help you with right now? I have made time available to help you."

Notes:

_____
_____
_____

Action Plan to Sustain Strengths

Specific

_____
_____

Measurable

_____
_____

Attainable

_____
_____

Realistic

_____
_____

Time-bound

_____
_____

Action Plan to Improve Weaknesses

Specific

_____
_____

Measurable

_____
_____

Attainable

_____
_____

Realistic

_____
_____

Time-bound

_____
_____

Topics to Discuss at Next One-on-One Meeting

TOPIC:	LEVEL OF DIFFICULTY:
	First floor (easy to implement)
	Second floor (moderately difficult to implement)
	Third floor (hard to implement)

IMPACT:	FOLLOW-UP:
	Immediate response necessary (before next 1:1)
	Moderate response (at next 1:1)
	Latent response (within six weeks)

Sample Rounding on Internal Departments

The purpose of this template is to provide a comprehensive tool for rounding with managers or directors of internal departments that support our department (housekeeping, maintenance, human resources, lab, radiology). This tool will help you identify interdepartmental wins and opportunities. Monthly rounding with various departmental managers or directors helps to build rapport in a proactive manner.

Sample Rounding on Internal Departments

Develop the Rounding Plan for Key Internal Customers

(Determine who in the department you will round with and the frequency; i.e., monthly or bimonthly.)

Leader name:_____Date: _____

Direct report name:_____Department:_____

Sample Impromptu Scripting for AIDET (Role Model; Studer, 2004)

Acknowledge	"I want you to know I appreciate the time you are taking out of your busy schedule to meet with me."
Introduce	"As you may know, my role in the organization is to ensure we have a healthy workplace environment." (Introduce your name and role if this is the first meeting.)
Duration	"Our one-on-one meeting will take approximately 15 minutes to one hour, depending on the acuity of the responses. I will ask you approximately seven questions that will help identify wins and opportunities between our departments."
Explanation	"The purpose of our meetings is to provide shared transparency. We will discuss rewards and recognition, as well as how we can improve current systems and processes. Please feel free to be upfront with me. Your opinion matters."
Thank you	"Thank you for taking time to talk with me. Your feedback is appreciated."

Healthy Workplace Environment

1. "Are there any systems or processes that do not meet your expectations?" (Circle)

    a. No—all systems and processes meet my expectations.

    b. Yes—please provide solutions on how to meet your expectations.

    _____
    _____

2. "Are there any systems or processes that exceed your expectations?"

    a. No—all systems and processes meet my expectations.

    b. Yes—please provide your rationale for why this exceeds your expectations.

    _____
    _____

Staff Rewards and Recognition

1. "Have any of my staff gone 'above and beyond' in their role?"

    Name _____

    Situation

    _____
    _____

    Action

    _____
    _____

    Response

    _____
    _____

2. "Have any providers in my department gone 'above and beyond' their role?"

    Name _____

    Situation

    _____
    _____

    Action

    _____
    _____

    Response

    _____
    _____

3. "Have you seen any other department go 'above and beyond' their role?"

   Name _____

   Situation

   _____
   _____

   Action

   _____
   _____

   Response

   _____
   _____

4. "Have any staff member(s) in other departments gone 'above and beyond' their role?"

   Name _____

   Situation

   _____
   _____

   Action

   _____
   _____

   Response

   _____
   _____

Coaching Questions

1. "We all experience difficult situations at different times. Do you have any at this time that I can address?"

    a. No issues at this time to be addressed.

    b. Yes—please provide details about the situation.

    Situation

    _____

    _____

    Action

    _____

    _____

    Response

    _____

    _____

    c. Use the TELL acronym to address tough issues or difficult conversations that you need to address.

    Tell or talk about the behavior.

    _____

    _____

    Explain why there is an issue.

    _____

    _____

Lead what is expected.

_____

_____

Learn the consequence.

_____

_____

Thank you.

"Thank you for meeting with me. Is there anything I can help you with right now? I have made time available to help you."

Notes:

_____

_____

_____

Action Plan to Sustain Strengths

Specific

_____

_____

Measurable

_____

_____

Attainable

_____

_____

Realistic

_____
_____

Time-bound

_____
_____

Action Plan to Improve Weaknesses

Specific

_____
_____

Measurable

_____
_____

Attainable

_____
_____

Realistic

_____
_____

Time-bound

_____
_____

Topics to Discuss at Next One-on-One Meeting

TOPIC:	LEVEL OF DIFFICULTY:
	First floor (easy to implement)
	Second floor (moderately difficult to implement)
	Third floor (hard to implement)
IMPACT:	**FOLLOW-UP:**
	Immediate response necessary (before next 1:1)
	Moderate response (at next 1:1)
	Latent response (within six weeks)

Reference

Studer, Q. (2004). *Hardwiring excellence: Purpose, worthwhile work, making a difference.* Studer Fire Starter Publishing.

B

Develop Your Own AIDET Worksheet

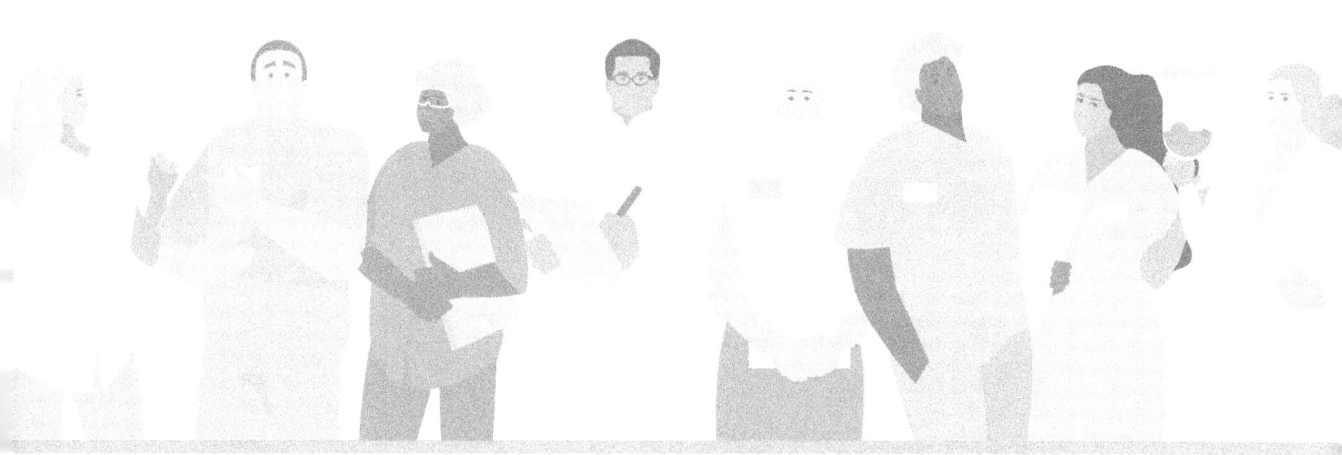

AIDET is an evidence-based communication model that provides a framework for communication with patients, families, and other healthcare providers. AIDET stands for:

- **A**cknowledge
- **I**ntroduce
- **D**uration
- **E**xplanation
- **T**hank you

This model is designed specifically to help gain the trust of others.

AIDET	EXAMPLES	PERSONALIZE IT
Acknowledge	Make patients and families feel welcome (e.g., smile).	
	Make patients and families feel comfortable (e.g., assess your body language).	
	Ask permission to enter a room.	
Introduce	Introduce yourself: Name/title: Years of experience/employment: Special training: Introduce others: Name/title: Years of experience/employment: Special training:	
Duration	Say how long the process, test, procedure, etc. will take.	
	Say when results will be back or when medications are due.	
	Say when the provider or nurse will arrive.	
	Say how long the referral process takes.	
	Say how long it will be before a physical assessment can be completed.	

Explanation	Explain the procedure or process and how the patient will obtain results.
	Explain what will take place using terms the patient and family can understand.
	Explain who is involved in providing the patient's care.
	Explain whether the process will cause pain or discomfort.
	Explain what will happen after the procedure is completed.
	Explain any post-procedure requirements.
	Offer to answer any questions, respond to concerns, or resolve any complaints.
	Note whether any equipment being used makes noise.
	Explain why you move patients (e.g., to prevent pressure ulcers).
	Explain why patients have food restrictions.
	Explain why you are closing the curtain or door (to ensure privacy).
Thank you	Tell patients you appreciate them and enjoyed working with them.
	Thank the family for entrusting you with the care of their loved one.
	Ask whether the patient or family has any final questions or concerns.

Adapted from the book Hardwiring Excellence: Purpose, Worthwhile Work, Making a Difference, *by Quint Studer.*

Index

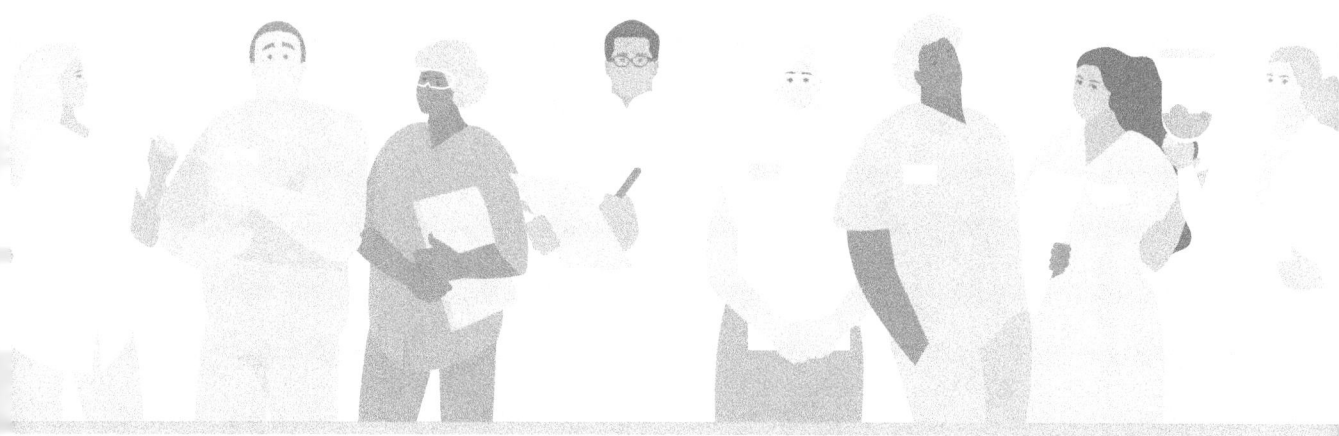

Note: Page references with an *f* are figures; page references with a *t* are tables.

A

ACCEPT, 223
accountability, 90
　versus ownership, 207
acknowledge (AIDET), 17, 18, 176–178
acknowledge differences (ACCEPT), 223
acronyms, scripting, 126–138
action
　CAR framework, 29–32, 59, 139
　STAR, 201
adaptation, 216
　to new organizational cultures, 226
AIDET communication framework, 17–18, 176–178
　worksheets, 271–272
American Association of Critical-Care Nurses (AACN), 192
American Heart Association's #CheckIt Challenge, 237
amiable social style, 7, 13–14
amiable styles, 10
amygdala, 64*f*
　fight-or-flight response, 101
　hijacking, 65, 129
analytical social styles, 7
analytical styles, 9, 11–12
anger, managing, 79
apologizing, 172, 173, 174–175
arm gestures, 44–45
Ash, Mary Kay, 4
ask questions (EMBRACE), 223
assessments
　behaviors, 224–226
　Hospital Consumer Assessment of Healthcare Providers and Systems (HCAHPS) survey, 185–187
　organizational culture, 224–226
　SBAR (situation, background, assessment, recommendation), 126, 127
　social styles, 8–11 (*see also* social styles)

B

backgrounds (SBAR), 126, 127
bad news, responding to, 132
be still and observe (EMBRACE), 223
bedside shift-change reporting, 180–181
behaviors, 211, 212
　assessments, 224–226
　communication, 222
　defining, 212–215
　social media, 240–245
　understanding, 215–224
being present, 104
being right, 91
belly-button rule, 55
belonging, 3*f*, 4
benefits
　of social media, 230
　of social styles, 11–16
BEST approach to conversations, 16–18, 16*f*, 119–120, 249. *See also* effective conversations
　body language, 18–20
　coaching, 156–162
　emotional intelligence (EI), 20–23
　scripting techniques, 23–25
best practices, research, 234–235
body language, 16, 17, 18–20, 33, 34–35, 105
　arm gestures, 44–45
　CAR framework, 59
　detecting honesty, 39–54
　hand gestures, 45–49
　handshakes, 50–51
　head gestures, 43–44
　improving messaging and interpretation, 55–61
　interpreting, 35–38
　legs and feet, 51–53
　mouth gestures, 39–43
　patient experience, 172, 173
　personal space, 54
　reading, 58
　social awareness, 74
　social styles, 36–38
brain processing emotions, 64*f*
brain-gut axis, 113–116
brainstorming, 200
breathing, 105
buy-in, motivating, 204–205

C

call to action (CAR framework), 29–32, 139
CAR framework, 29–32, 59
    coaching, 157–158
    patient experience, 187–188
    scripting, 138–140
celebrate diversity (ACCEPT), 223
Centers for Medicare & Medicaid Services (CMS), 4, 249
challenging situations, scripting, 125t–126t
change
    embracing, 193–195
    leadership, 193–195
    management, 193 (*see also* managing)
    organizational, 225
chats, X (formally Twitter), 232–233. *See also* social media
chemicals, selfish, 113
Cleveland Clinic, 213
cliques, 222
coaching, 141, 142
    BEST approach to conversations, 156–162
    CAR framework, 157–158
    curiosity and, 148–149
    emotions, 151–152
    framing conversations, 150–151
    hard-to-have conversations, 142–156
    leadership training, 143–147
    listening skills, 180
    overcoming conversational traps, 152–155
    reflection, 155–156
    TELL framework, 158–163
collaboration, 70
    networking with social media, 230–233
commitment, lack of, 194
committees, establishing key, 197–204
common sense, 4, 5–8
communication, 2, 248–251
    AIDET communication framework, 17–18, 176–178
    bedside shift-change reporting, 180–181
    behaviors, 222
    benefits of social styles, 11–16
    common sense, 5–8
    discharge phone calls, 182
    effective conversations, 16–18
    Five Rights of Communication Safety, 30–31
    hourly rounds, 179–180
    improving, 9, 74
    integrating teach-back into, 25–28
    interaction styles, 6–8
    Maslow's hierarchy of needs theory model, 3–5, 3f
    mindful conversations (*see* mindful conversations)
    nonverbal, 35 (*see also* body language)
    patient experience, 176–188
    responding to bad news, 132
    science behind, 111–116
    scripting, 125–126 (*see also* scripting)
    skills, 74
    social styles, 8–11 (*see also* social styles)
    strategies, 248
    whiteboards, 178–179
components of effective conversations, 17
conclusions, jumping to, 55
condescending, avoiding being, 155
conflict resolution, 138
connections, 2. *See also* communication
consideration
    CAR framework, 29–32
    how you present yourself (EMBRACE), 223
    for others (ACCEPT), 223
controlling
    emotions, 75–83
    power and, 215–216
    taking control, 91
    tone, 103
conversations. *See also* communication
    BEST approach to, 119–120
    coaching (*see* coaching)
    common sense, 5–8
    conversation sandwiches, 152
    effective, 16–18
    hard-to-have, 142–156
    improving, 100
    integrating teach-back into, 25–28
    mindful, 97, 98–100 (*see also* mindful conversations)
    overcoming conversational traps, 152–155
    walking away, 153
copycats, 58
core competencies, leadership training, 143
cortisol, 65

COVID-19, 2
Cuddy, Amy, 119
cultures
    behaviors, 212 (*see also* behaviors)
    organizational, 211, 212 (*see also* organizational culture)
curiosity, 148–149

D

deception, 59, 216. *See also* honesty, detecting
decision trees, 139*f*
detecting honesty, 39–54
    arm gestures, 44–45
    hand gestures, 45–49
    handshakes, 50–51
    head gestures, 43–44
    legs and feet, 51–53
    mouth gestures, 39–43
    personal space, 54
diets, 118
disadvantages of social media, 238–239
disappointment, managing, 82
DISC (Dominant, Influential, Steady, and Conscientious) assessment, 8
discharge follow-up, 202
dislike, managing, 82
disrupting emotional cycles, 67
distractions, eliminating, 105
dominant handshakes, 50
dopamine, 112
Doximity, 231. *See also* social media
Dr. Mike's YouTube Channel, 238
dramatic, avoiding being, 155
driver styles, 9, 12–13
driving social style, 7
due diligence, social media, 240–245
duration (AIDET), 17, 18, 176–178
Dweck, Carol, 110

E

eating right, 118
education. *See also* training
    leadership, 203
    social media, 235–238
effective conversations, 16–18. *See also* conversations
    body language, 18–20
    components of, 17
    emotional intelligence (EI), 20–23
    guiding principles for, 29–32
    scripting techniques, 23–25
EMBRACE, 223
embracing change, 193–195
Emotional and Social Competency Inventory (ESCI), 70
emotional competency (EC), 128
    impact of, 69–70
    improving, 73–91
    need for, 68–69
emotional intelligence (EI), 16, 17, 20–23, 63, 64–66
    collaboration, 70
    impact of, 69–70
    improving, 73–91
    leadership skills, 83–90
    measuring, 70
    Myers-Briggs Type Indicator (MBTI), 71–72
    need for emotional competency (EC), 68–69
    Oz principle, 90–91
    scripting, 128–138
    understanding, 66–72
    working with emotions, 67–68
Emotional Quotient Inventory 2.0 (EQ-i 2.0), 70
emotions
    brain processing, 64*f*
    coaching, 151–152
    controlling, 75–83
    negative, 112
    working with, 67–68
empathetic response (SPIKES), 183–185
empathy, 66, 68, 105
    increasing, 9
empathy (ACCEPT), 223
empowering women, 4
encourage (EMBRACE), 223
enculturation, 225
endorphins, 112
engagement (EMBRACE), 223
enteric nervous system (ENS), 114
episodes, 66. *See also* emotional intelligence (EI)
establishing key committees, 197–204
esteem, 3*f*, 4
ethics, social media, 239–240

etiquette
    cultural behavior, 217
    rules of, 149
exercise, 118
explain/explore perspectives (TELL framework), 23, 26, 27
explanation (AIDET), 18, 176–178
expressive social styles, 7, 14–16
expressive styles, 10
Extroversion-Introversion (MBTI), 71
extrovert, sensor, thinker, and judger (ESTJ), 72
eye contact, 58. *See also* body language
eye gestures, interpreting, 37*t*–38*t*

F

Facebook, 231, 232. *See also* social media
facial expressions, 34, 58. *See also* body language
facts, sticking to, 154
fight-or-flight response, 65, 101
Figure 1, 231. *See also* social media
Five Rights of Communication Safety, 30–31
fixed mindsets, 110
formal leadership training, 143–147
formality, 217
formulas, Question-Wait-Question (QWQ), 75
fostering relationships, 68*t*–69*t*
fostering trust, 226
framing coaching conversations, 150–151
frustration, 78
full-time equivalent (FTE), 69

G

Gallup survey, 199
Geisinger Health System, 213
gender, hierarchy and, 218–220
generalizations, 154
generating ideas, 204
gestures
    arm, 44–45
    eye, 37*t*–38*t*
    hand, 45–49
    head, 43–44

improving body language, 55–61
    interpreting, 35
    legs and feet, 51–53
    mouth, 39–43
    personal space, 54
    scripting, 124 (*see also* scripting)
Gigerenzer, Gerd, 114
Golden Rule, 138
growth mindsets, 110
guidelines
    for effective conversations, 29–32
    social media, 240–245
Gut Feelings: The Intelligence of the Unconscious (Gigerenzer), 114

H

hand gestures, 45–49
handshakes, 50–51
hard-to-have conversations, 142–156
head gestures, 43–44
health illiteracy, 25
Health Insurance Portability and Accountability Act (HIPAA), 240
healthy workplace environments (HWEs), 191, 192–193
    embracing change, 193–195
    inspiring others, 226
    leadership, 195–207
    TELL framework, 196–197
HEARD (hear, empathize, apologize, resolve, diagnose), 172–173, 249
hierarchy
    and gender, 218–220
    of needs, 3–5, 3*f*
hiring practices, 200–201
honesty, detecting, 39–54
hormones, stress, 65
Hospital Consumer Assessment of Healthcare Providers and Systems (HCAHPS) survey, 4, 5, 185–187, 249
hourly rounds, 179–180
hurry up and wait, 193–194

I

ideas, generating, 204
impromptu scripts, 124, 125–126. *See also* scripting
improving
    behaviors, 224–226
    body language messaging and interpretation, 55–61
    communication, 9, 74
    conversations, 98, 100 (*see also* mindful conversations)
    emotional competency (EC), 73–91
    emotional intelligence (EI), 73–91
    leadership skills, 83–90
    organizational culture, 224–226
    outcomes, 116–120
    patient experience, 165, 166–167 (*see also* patient experience)
    relationships, 9
    teamwork, 9
inconsistencies, noticing, 55
informal leadership training, 143–147
information resources, social media, 233–235
inspiring others, 226
instincts, fight-or-flight response, 101
integrating
    arm gestures, 44–45
    teach-back into conversations, 25–28
intention, understanding, 103
interaction styles, 6–8
internal motivation, 66
interpreting
    body language, 35–38 (*see also* body language)
    detecting honesty, 39–54
    eye gestures, 37*t*–38*t*
    gestures, 35
    head gestures, 43–44
    improving body language, 55–61
interprofessional coaching, 141, 142. *See also* coaching
introduce (AIDET), 17, 18, 176–178
invitation (SPIKES), 183–185

J

Judging-Perceiving (MTBI), 71

K

Kaiser Permanente, 213
key committees, establishing, 197–204
knowledge
    deficits, 194
    SPIKES, 183–185

L

lack
    of commitment, 194
    of practice, 194
leadership
    accountability versus ownership, 207
    change, 193–195
    discharge follow-up, 202
    establishing key committees, 197–204
    generating ideas, 204
    healthy workplace environments (HWEs), 195–207
    hiring practices, 200–201
    improving skills, 83–90
    motivation, 204–205
    neuroleadership, 111, 112
    physician and staff engagement, 203–204
    rewards and recognition, 199–200
    training, 143–147, 203
    transformation, 205–207
    transformation rounding, 202
    welcoming new recruits, 202–203
LEARN (listen, empathize, ask, recognize, notice), 128–129
legal issues, social media and, 239–240
legs and feet gestures, 51–53
leveraging shared values (TELL framework), 23, 26, 27
LinkedIn, 231. *See also* social media
listening skills, 98, 105, 180
listening to perspectives (TELL framework), 23, 26, 27
love, 3*f*, 4
lying, detecting, 39. *See also* honesty

M

majority rules, common sense and, 5
managing
    anger, 79
    conflicts, 138
    disappointment, 82
    dislike, 82
    emotions, 66
    relationships, 74, 136–138
    routines, 118
Maslow's hierarchy of needs theory model, 3–5, 3*f*
Mayer-Salovey-Caruso Emotional Intelligence Test (MSCEIT), 70
Mayo Clinic, 212
    Facebook Live sessions, 237
meanings of gestures, 37. *See also* body language; gestures; interpreting
    arm gestures, 45*t*
    hand gestures, 46*t*–49*t*
    handshakes, 51*t*
    head gestures, 43*t*–44*t*
    legs and feet gestures, 52*t*–53*t*
    mouth gestures, 42*t*–43*t*
    personal space, 54*t*
measuring
    emotional intelligence (EI), 70
    patient experience, 185–187
    success, 111
MedEdWorld, 231. *See also* social media
meditation, 101. *See also* mindful conversations
mental models, 109, 110–111
mind over matter, 109, 110–111
    brain-gut axis, 113–116
    improving outcomes, 116–120
    neurotransmitters, 112–113
    science behind communication, 111–116
mindful conversations, 97, 98–100
    being present, 104
    improving conversations, 100
    negative emotions, 101–102
    overview of mindfulness, 99–100
    self-acceptance, 102
    understanding intention, 103
Mindful Leader Summit (2022), 104

Mindfulness-Based Stress Reduction (MBSR), 101
Mindset: The New Psychology of Success (Dweck), 110
mindsets
    adjusting, 105
    fixed, 110
    growth, 110
models
    Maslow's hierarchy of needs theory, 3–5, 3*f*
    Social Styles Model, 8*f*
    standards of behavior (EMBRACE), 223
moment, remaining in, 105. *See also* mindful conversations
moods, 102. *See also* emotional intelligence (EI)
motivation, 55, 68, 73
    leadership, 204–205
    patients to care for themselves, 182–183
    scripting, 134
mouth, detecting honesty, 39–43
mutual handshakes, 50, 50*f*
Myers-Briggs Type Indicator (MBTI), 71–72

N

naughty bits rule, 55
needs
    for emotional competency (EC), 68–69
    hierarchy of, 3–5
negative cultures, 194
negative emotions, 67, 112. *See also* emotional intelligence (EI)
    mindful conversations, 101–102
neocortex, 64*f*
networking with social media, 230–233
neurodivergent, 114, 115
neuroleadership, 111, 112
neuroscience, mindful conversations and, 101
neurotransmitters, 112–113
neurotypical, 114
nonverbal communication, 35. *See also* body language
nurses
    Facebook for, 231–232
    networking with social media, 230–233

O

open-ended questions, 24, 105, 127f
    coaching conversations, 150
organizational change, 225
organizational culture, 211, 212
    assessments, 224–226
    communication, 222
    defining, 212–215
    understanding, 215–224
outcomes, improving, 116–120
overcoming conversational traps, 152–155
overthinkers, 115
ownership, accountability versus, 207
oxytocin, 113
Oz principle, 90–91

P

pain, 112
pandemics, 2. *See also* COVID-19
paraphrasing, 105
patient experience
    AIDET communication framework, 176–178
    bedside shift-change reporting, 180–181
    CAR framework, 187–188
    communication, 176–188
    discharge phone calls, 182
    hourly rounds, 179–180
    improving, 165, 166–167
    measuring, 185–187
    motivation to care for themselves, 182–183
    perception (is reality), 167
    SPIKES, 183–185
    strategies, 167–175
    whiteboards, 178–179
perceive the environment (ACCEPT), 223
perception
    SPIKES, 183–185
    of time, 218
personal space, 36, 54, 58
personal styles, 6, 7
phone calls, discharge, 182
phrases
    for empathy, 135t
    for relationship management, 137t
    for social awareness, 135t

physical pain, 112
physician and staff engagement, 203–204
physiological needs, 3f
planning, 124. *See also* scripting
power
    and control, 215–216
    of the pause, 75
    posing, 119f
practice, lack of, 194
preferences, styles, 10f
prefrontal cortex (PFC), 65
present, being, 104
Press Ganey Associates, 250
principles
    for effective conversations, 29–32
    Oz principle, 90–91
privacy, 240
proactive statements, 132
processing emotions, 64. *See also* emotional intelligence
professionals, networking with social media, 230–233
promotion, social media, 235–238

Q

Question-Wait-Question (QWQ) formula, 75
questions
    coaching conversations, 150
    open-ended, 24, 105, 127f

R

reactive statements, 132
reading body language, 58
recognition, 199–200
recommendations (SBAR), 126, 127
reflect (EMBRACE), 223
regulating emotions, 66
relationships
    communication skills, 251 (*see also* communication)
    emotional intelligence (EI) and collaboration, 70
    fostering, 68t–69t
    improving, 9
    managing, 74, 136–138
relaxation, 101. *See also* mindful conversations

reports
    bedside shift-change reporting, 180–181
    Hospital Consumer Assessment of Healthcare Providers and Systems (HCAHPS) survey, 185–187
research, best practices, 234–235
ResearchGate, 231. *See also* social media
respect, showing, 225
responding to bad news, 132
result (STAR), 201
return on investment (ROI), 29–32, 139
rewards, 199–200
rights, Five Rights of Communication Safety, 30–31
Rock, David, 111
routines, managing, 118
rules
    belly-button, 55
    of etiquette, 149
    naughty bits, 55

S

safety, 3*f*
    Five Rights of Communication Safety, 30–31
sample rounding templates
    internal departments, 262–269
    transformational, 253–262
SBAR (situation, background, assessment, recommendation), 126, 127, 249
science
    behind communication, 111–116
    brain-gut axis, 113–116
    neurotransmitters, 112–113
scripting, 16, 17, 23–25
    acronyms, 126–138
    CAR framework, 138–140
    challenging situations, 125*t*–126*t*
    definition of, 123, 124
    emotional intelligence (EI), 128–138
    empathy, 134–136
    Hospital Consumer Assessment of Healthcare Providers and Systems (HCAHPS) survey, 185–187
    impromptu scripts, 125–126
    motivation, 134
    relationship management, 136–138
    responding to bad news, 132
    self-awareness, 128–129
    self-regulation, 129–134
self-acceptance, 102
self-actualization, 3*f*, 4
self-awareness, 66, 68, 73
    scripting, 128–129
self-regulation, 66, 68, 73
    scripting, 129–134
selfish chemicals, 113
Sensing-Intuition (MBTI), 71
SERMO, 231. *See also* social media
serotonin, 113
setting (SPIKES), 183–185
sexual harassment, 56–57
sharing stories, 226
Shriver, Maria, 75
situation (STAR), 201
situations (SBAR), 126, 127
Six Seconds Emotional Intelligence Test (SEI), 70
skills
    communication, 74
    leadership, 83–90
    listening, 98, 105
    managing conflicts, 138
    social, 66
sly foxes, 153, 154
social awareness, 74
social media, 229, 230
    benefits of, 230
    disadvantages of, 238–239
    due diligence, 240–245
    as education/promotion tool, 235–238
    ethics, 239–240
    information resources, 233–235
    legal issues, 239–240
    networking with, 230–233
social skills, 66, 68
social styles, 6, 7
    amiable social style, 13–14
    analytical styles, 11–12
    benefits of, 11–16
    body language, 36–38 (*see also* body language)
    communication, 8–11
    driver styles, 12–13
    expressive social style, 14–16
    fostering relationships, 68*t*–69*t*

Social Styles Model, 8, 8f
socialization, 225
speaking. *See also* communication
    mindful conversations, 98 (*see also* mindful conversations)
    personal space, 58
    responding to bad news, 132
    scripting, 125–126 (*see also* scripting)
SPIKES, 183–185
standards (HWEs), 192, 193
STAR (situation, task, action, result), 201
statements
    proactive, 132
    reactive, 132
stories, sharing, 226
strategies
    communication, 248
    patient experience, 167–175
    SPIKES, 183–185
stress hormones, 65
Studer Group, 213
styles
    interaction, 6–8
    personal, 6, 7
    preferences, 10f
    social, 6, 7, 8–11 (*see also* social styles)
    Social Styles Model, 8f
submissive handshakes, 50
success
    cultural behaviors, 214
    measuring, 111
suffering, 112
surveys
    Gallup survey, 199
    Hospital Consumer Assessment of Healthcare Providers and Systems (HCAHPS) survey, 185–187

TELL framework, 23, 26, 27, 40–41. *See also* communication
    coaching, 144–147, 158–163
    healthy workplace environments (HWEs), 196–197
    patient experience, 174–175
    scripting, 130–131
    sexual harassment, 56–57
templates
    internal departments, 262–269
    transformational, 253–262
testing emotional intelligence (EI), 70. *See also* measuring
thalamus, 64f
thank you (AIDET), 18, 176–178
Thinking-Feeling (MTBI), 71
time
    perception of, 218
    and place to talk (TELL framework), 23, 26, 27
time-sensitive decisions, 139f
    decision trees, 139f
tips and tools, 16, 17. *See also* effective conversations
tolerate only respect (ACCEPT), 223
tone, taming, 103
tools, social media, 235–238
training
    leadership, 203
    leadership skills, 143–147
transformational leadership, 205–207
transformational rounding, 202
trust
    building, 2 (*see also* communication)
    fostering, 226
    trusting instincts, 58
Tuckman, Bruce, 199
3WITH method, 127, 127f, 128, 129
2BROKE, 39

T

talking, 24. *See also* communication
task (STAR), 201
teach-back into conversations, integrating, 25–28
teamwork, 9. *See also* committees, establishing key; leadership

U

undermining
    others, 155
    yourself, 154
understanding
    behaviors, 215–224

body language, 35–38 (*see also* body language)
emotional intelligence (EI), 66–72
increasing, 9
intention, 103
organizational culture, 215–224
showing, 105

V

Varshavski, Mikhail, 238
victimization, 90–91
visual cortex, 64*f*
Voltaire, 4

W

walking away, 153
welcoming new recruits, 202–203
whiteboards, 178–179
women, empowering, 4
words, motivational, 134*t*
work ethics, 222
worksheets (AIDET), 271–272
World Health Organization's (WHO) X updates, 237
worry, 78–79

X

X (formally Twitter), 231. *See also* social media
    chats, 232–233

www.ingramcontent.com/pod-product-compliance
Lightning Source LLC
Chambersburg PA
CBHW060336010526
44117CB00017B/2848